Supporting Parents with Alzheimer's:

Your parents took care of you, now how do you take care of them?

Supporting Parents with Alzheimer's:

Your parents took care of you, now how do you take care of them?

Tanya Lee Howe

Self-Counsel Press
(a division of)
International Self-Counsel Press Ltd.
USA   Canada

Self-Counsel Press acknowledges the financial support of the Government of Canada through the Canada Book Fund (CBF) for our publishing activities.

Printed in Canada.

First edition: 2013; Reprinted: 2013

Library and Archives Canada Cataloguing in Publication

Howe, Tanya Lee

Supporting parents with alzheimer's / Tanya Lee Howe.

ISBN 978-1-77040-149-5

1. Alzheimer's disease — Patients — Care. 2. Alzheimer's disease — Patients — Family relationships. I. Title.

RC523.H69 2013   616.8'31   C2012-903079-1

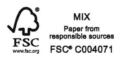

MIX
Paper from
responsible sources
FSC® C004071

Self-Counsel Press
(a division of)
International Self-Counsel Press Ltd.

Bellingham, WA	North Vancouver, BC
USA	Canada

Contents

2 The Memory Book

3 Alzheimer's Planner for Caregivers

Samples

Notice to Readers

Laws are constantly changing. Every effort is made to keep this publication as current as possible. However, the author, the publisher, and the vendor of this book make no representations or warranties regarding the outcome or the use to which the information in this book is put and are not assuming any liability for any claims, losses, or damages arising out of the use of this book. The reader should not rely on the author or the publisher of this book for any professional advice. Please be sure that you have the most recent edition.

Dedication

First and foremost, I dedicate this book to Mom. I would not have been able to write it without your support and willingness to share your story.

I am so grateful to my wonderful sister-in-law, Sheila Janzen. She was the one who came up with the original idea for the *Alzheimer's Planner for Caregivers* (see Chapter 3). I would have never been as organized if it wasn't for her advice and help. Even though Sheila hates writing, she spent countless hours writing notes on Mom's behavior. Thank you to Sheila, Shawn, Ashleigh, Kaiden, and Myranda for opening your home to Mom.

Thank you to Cecelia De Smit for being a true friend to Mom and to our family. Your visits with Mom have been valuable to her well-being such as the many laughs and memories you both share from six decades of friendship. Sheila and I also thank you for taking Mom when we needed a weekend each month to give ourselves some well-needed self-care.

To my husband, Darren Howe, thank you for all the things you do for me and my family. You are the glue that holds me together. I have never met another man who has your patience and understanding. Also, your adventures give me lots to laugh about when I'm feeling blue!

Thank you to my dad for listening to me when I just needed to vent. You've always been there for me and I appreciate everything you do for me. To my stepmom, Carol, thank you for being a wonderful second mom to me. I'm also grateful for your help with my research; you have sent me valuable information that has contributed to this book.

I also want to say thanks to Jocelyn Rawleigh for putting her life on hold to help me promote a cause. We both have lists of "100 Things to Do before We Die" and I'm happy that a couple of the items on our lists just happen to coincide!

Thanks to Eileen "Madam Editrix" Velthuis for helping me to make my dreams come true. You have given me wonderful advice as both a friend and business associate. I can fly again and that is because of you!

Thank you to Self-Counsel Press, and especially Richard Day and Diana Douglas, for publishing two books with topics that meant a lot to me to be able to share with the world.

Thank you Dr. Derman (and his wonderful staff) for your kind words, and for being a doctor who treats his patients with respect and care. I wish every person was lucky enough to have such a wonderful doctor.

Thank you to Conny Schipper, Janet Cook, Heather Mueller, Christine Ratkai, Travis Asplund, Lisa Barrett, and Lynn Crackel for taking the time to answer my questions and to donate words to these pages. Thank you to Trudy Curtis for making me laugh on the days when I thought laughter wasn't possible.

Finally, to my dearest Orph, for making me realize life is too short to waste. I miss you buddy.

Author's Note

"Every 72 seconds someone in America develops Alzheimer's."

— ALZHEIMER'S ASSOCIATION

Alzheimer's disease (AD) is one of the most common forms of dementia. There is no known cause or cure for this progressive and terminal brain disorder. I have observed what a heartbreaking disease it is by watching my mother go through memory loss, confusion and disorientation, fear, and impaired judgment. Her personality has moved from vibrant and independent to a feeling of sadness and dependence. With Sheila, my sister-in-law, and the rest of the family's help, we have been able to increase Mom's happiness during the progression of the disease.

My grandma was first diagnosed when she was 78 years old. I know my grandma showed signs earlier but I don't remember how much earlier. My mother was officially diagnosed at 68 years old. The first time I noticed the signs with my mom was when she was 59.

In the mid-1980s, my grandma began the slow crawl into AD. At that time my mom struggled to get information about the disease, at least nowadays there is more information for helping a person with AD. However, in my opinion, not enough has been done in the last 30 years to find a cause *and* cure for AD. If something isn't discovered soon, the chances of my brother and I having AD in the next 20 to 30 years is a very real possibility.

Estimates vary, but experts suggest that more than 5.1 million Americans and 500,000 Canadians have AD. According to the article "Alzheimer's Unlocked" (*Time*, October 25, 2010), by Alice Park:

"'We spend $5.6 billion a year funding cancer studies, $1 billion a year on heart disease ... and $500 million to study Alzheimer's,' said Dr. Ronald Petersen, director of the Mayo Clinic Alzheimer's Disease Research Center.' Yet what is going to get most of us in the next few years is Alzheimer's.'"

Two years later, in a news release on May 12, 2012, it was announced that President Obama's administration had presented the National Plan to Address Alzheimer's Disease (aspe.hhs.gov/daltcp/napa/NatlPlan. pdf). The plan includes making additional funding available to support research, provide clinicians with more education, and spread public awareness about the disease. There will also be funding for new research projects and easier access to information for support caregivers.

If your loved one is showing signs of AD, please learn as much as you can about the disease and spread awareness. The more people who know about it means more funding will go toward this disease and a cure will be found. In the United States, contact the Alzheimer's Association (www.alz.org); and in Canada, the Alzheimer Society (www.alzheimer. ca) to see what you can do to help fight Alzheimer's disease.

This book is written from the research and experience of our family. Every situation is different, but I hope that some of the information in this book will help you and your family on your journey with your loved one.

Introduction

"Alzheimer's disease can be a hard journey, but it can also be filled with many special moments you can share with your loved one."

— UNKNOWN

> You can download free worksheets and checklists to create your own *Alzheimer's Planner for Caregivers*, as well as get links to additional resources by going to this address with your computer web browser:
>
> http://self-counsel.com/updates/alz/check13.html

This book is designed to help those moving a parent with Alzheimer's Disease (or with another form of dementia) into a family member's home. My research is based on talking with professionals (e.g., doctors, the Alzheimer Society, nurses) and other families in similar situations; it is also based on the steps our family took to move my mother, who was in the mid-stage of Alzheimer's disease (AD) and was rapidly moving toward the advanced stage at the time we stepped in to help.

I believe moving Mom home has given her another year with family as opposed to having to move straight into a long-term care home. This book will give you an understanding of what we have done to help work with the disease and to make life as comfortable as we can for her before the next step of moving her into long-term care. We have given her a quality of life she wouldn't have had in her former home. She needs someone around 24 hours a day, seven days a week, which has been a struggle at times but the good memories the family has gathered during this time has been worth it.

It's a personal decision that family members need to discuss before moving the parent. I'm fortunate to have a sister-in-law, Sheila, who feels like a blood sister to me. This experience has made our families grow closer, which is something Mom has always wanted for us.

In our situation, my house does not include an extra bedroom; instead, Sheila offered her and my brother's home. My oldest niece, Myranda, had moved away, so they had a room to spare. I have to commend my sister-in-law because she stepped up without hesitation.

Our journey with Mom began in the summer of 2011. Mom drove from Saskatoon, Saskatchewan, to Lethbridge, Alberta, for a surprise visit. It had been a couple years since I had seen her, which was not unusual for us — we've always been close by phone. Her surprise visit wasn't unusual either because over the years, when she wanted to go for a short vacation she would just hop in her car and show up on our doorstep.

Mom was two hours late when I received a frantic phone call from her. She told me she was at a corner store, but when I looked at the call display on my phone, it named another store. I calmly asked her to put the manager on the phone, which turned out to be someone I knew. The manager kept an eye on her as she paced in front of the store until I got there.

When I drove up to the store, she didn't recognize me until I said, "Mom." Relief washed over her face and she rushed to my passenger car door trying to open it. "Mom, where's your car?" She looked at me confused and attempted to open the passenger door again. Again, I asked her where her car was. Her face showed a moment of clarity and then she marched across the parking lot to her car, and then she drove behind me to my home. She was slightly confused and anxious for the rest of the evening.

This book describes the steps and information Sheila and I had to learn in order to help Mom with the transition of moving. It was hard for all of us because we didn't have a clue about what to do or who to contact. It was so overwhelming for me, because the person I turned to for advice was now depending on me to give her advice and make decisions for her. Being that I've never had children, I knew very little about taking care of someone who was dependent. It is a huge responsibility but also an honor that Mom trusted us to take care of her during this time.

While this book was mainly written for sons and daughters looking for answers on how to deal with their parents who may now be going into early to mid-stage AD or dementia; in this world of blended families more and more adults are having to help uncles, aunts, stepparents, and even elderly siblings with cognitive impairments. AD doesn't affect just seniors; there are cases of people in their 30s, 40s, and 50s with the disease as well.

When a person you love begins to lose the ability to think properly, remember what happened yesterday (or even an hour ago), formulate ideas, or concentrate on a simple task, what do you do? How do you convince someone he or she can no longer take care of himself or herself? Chapter 1 discusses signs that your loved one needs someone to step in and help him or her. It also includes information on how to talk with the person about the move.

There are many good books dedicated solely to the topics of power of attorney, enduring power of attorney, living wills, and health-care directives; however, you will need to know some basics about these important documents. Chapters 1 and 5 include information about the necessity of having this paperwork in place before you begin moving your elderly relative.

We discovered the value of the Memory Book from Mom. She had been writing in memory books for the previous seven years. It wasn't so much a journal, but a book to keep track of what she was doing from day to day. She included shopping lists, trips to the doctor, social events, and sometimes her mood swings and fears. When we mentioned this to her new doctor in Alberta, he said, "You have inspired me to encourage my other patients with memory issues to create their own memory books." This in turn, gave Mom a big boost of confidence knowing she had inspired a doctor. (I owe Dr. Derman a big thank you for all the kindness, patience, and understanding he has given to both Mom and me.) Chapter 2 goes into the benefits of having your loved one create his or her own Memory Book.

Sheila and I divided our caretaking duties, but we kept all the information in one book that we passed back and forth between us when we took Mom to different appointments. We called this the *Alzheimer's Planner for Caregivers*. This was one of the most important tools for us to stay organized. It also helped us to reduce our caregiver stress. (See Chapter 3 for more information.)

You will find in the following pages help for transitioning the person with AD to your home. There are many reasons your parent may need to move in with you. In some areas there are long waiting lists for long-term care homes, and in some situations, the person cannot afford to move into a care home so the only option is to move the person into a family member's home. The biggest challenge is helping the person adjust to the new living environment (see Chapter 4), but it can also be a big adjustment for the caretakers.

What you and I deem organized and logical will not always be so with a person suffering from AD. You may find important paperwork stashed in books, boxes, kitchen cupboards, or nowhere at all, so where do you begin? What do you do with all the stuff in storage or the knick-knacks that won't fit in the new place? Chapter 4 discusses the problems and solutions for going through someone's personal items.

There are many important government agencies you will need to contact as well as doctors and other experts who understand AD. If your parent is no longer fit to drive, how do you approach this topic? This can be a touchy subject because most people consider a license as a form of independence. Chapter 5 will take you through the steps to dealing with these important topics.

Chapter 6 discusses your loved one's finances, how to find all the accounts, organizing the bills and paying debts, and closing or transferring accounts.

Chapter 7 discusses some ways to help your parent cope with the disease. As a caregiver, you will need to understand AD as best you can in order to help your parent go through the progression of it. You may find your parent becomes difficult when it comes to bathing or changing his or her clothes. You will find tips in Chapter 7 to help you with difficult behavior.

You will need to find meaningful activities at the appropriate skill level for your relative with AD. Chapter 8 will give you suggestions of things to do with your loved one as well as solo activities. It is important that your parent is socially and physically active, which will help him or her be happier.

This book does not cover later stages of elder care, such as removing the elderly person from a long-term care home or abuses in a long-term care home environment. However, Chapter 9 discusses the complex issue of removing your relative from a bad home environment such as an abusive spouse or partner, whether it is verbal, mental, or physical abuse. When you are dealing with a victim with such a delicate frame of mind, removing him or her from a familiar place is not an easy task.

Chapter 10 discusses self-care for the caretaker. It's not always easy inviting a relative to live in your home. There will be a period of adjustment. Depending on how far advanced the cognitive impairment is, it may be necessary that the person never be left on his or her own. So how do you make time for yourself? You will need to learn to avoid caregiver burn out. If you can't take care of yourself, it is extremely hard to properly care for someone else.

What I have found during this journey with Mom, Sheila, and the rest of our family is that the good moments we have are cherished more now than they have ever been. Memories are repeated over and over, but I don't mind hearing Mom's stories again and again. They make her happy, which makes me happy. I wish you all the best on your journey with your loved one, and I hope this book helps you with the transition.

CHAPTER 1

Moving Your Parent into Your Home

"In just five years, as many as 50 percent more Canadians and their families could be facing Alzheimer's disease or another form of dementia."

— ALZHEIMER SOCIETY OF CANADA (2009)

Until Mom's visit in August, even though I had seen the signs many years earlier, I kept thinking we always had "one more year" until the moving topic needed to be discussed. I struggled with whether or not it would be right to move Mom away from the life she had known for the previous 16 years.

Unfortunately, within the last five or so years she had isolated herself from her friends, quit her job, and mainly stayed at home with her two dogs and boyfriend. Isolation was the way she coped with the disease, which saved her from feeling embarrassed in public.

After her visit to Alberta, my sister-in-law, Sheila, and I drove back to Saskatoon with Mom. We sat down and discussed with her and her boyfriend that it was time she moved home with us. She needed a strong family support network to help her. Her boyfriend clearly couldn't cope with her changing moods and her new "odd" habits and he didn't understand that she needed someone around 24 hours a day, seven days a week.

He mentioned how he had recently come into the house to find a cabbage burning in a pot on the stove. Mom had forgotten to put water in the pot and then she had completely forgotten she was cooking anything at all. She had gone off to do something else and didn't even notice the smoke billowing from the kitchen.

We made plans to come back in a couple of weeks to talk to her doctor and find out the best way to go about the move. When we returned, Mom was suffering from shingles. We took her to the doctor and discovered that Mom had been to the doctor twice the week before. The doctor didn't understand why Mom returned a second time (and now a third time with us) when she had already been given medication for the shingles. As we talked to the doctor, we discovered she didn't know that Mom had Alzheimer's disease (AD). Mom had told us she was on pills for AD and had already been diagnosed; however, she hadn't been prescribed pills or diagnosed.

The doctor learned from our visit about Mom's situation and in the end the doctor said, "I realize after this visit with you, the family, that I need to get to know my patients better." This is a major problem nowadays, there are not enough doctors for patients, which makes it hard for doctors to really get to know their patients due to lack of time.

I cannot stress enough that when you take over the care of your parent, you need to keep on top of all medical situations. You need to get to know the doctors, nurses, and others in the medical profession and get them to know your parent. Even though this book isn't about long-term care, when your parent goes into a care home someday, you still need to stay on top of everything that concerns your loved one; otherwise, he or she may get lost in the system.

We were told that if Mom was to stay in Saskatoon, it may be up to a year until she was able to see a Geriatric Specialist. Mom's general practitioner doctor said that considering the circumstances with Mom, she should go home with her family because we could provide a better network of help for her. The doctor suggested to help Mom with the transition that she come stay with us for three weeks, return to Saskatoon for three weeks, and then back to our place for another three weeks.

We returned a couple of weeks later to gather Mom and her items. When we arrived, we discovered the shingles had spread and they had become severely inflamed. We immediately took her to the hospital, where she was diagnosed with the worst case of shingles the doctor had ever seen.

We took her home to Alberta the next day and for the next three weeks we nursed her back to health. We weren't set up for the Alberta medical yet so there was a lot of medical care we couldn't access without paying for it. The brunt of the care fell to our family. At the end of the three weeks, we decided to not follow the doctor's suggestion of moving her back and forth for the next few months. We felt that moving her back and forth would cause her more stress and confusion, which is not good for someone suffering from AD.

This chapter provides you with the first steps of moving your parent into your home. Hopefully in your situation, you don't have to move your parent a long distance. If you are lucky, it is a matter of moving your parent from his or her home to your home within the same city as you.

1. Signs Your Parent Can No Longer Cope on His or Her Own

The signs your parent is not coping well living on his or her own may be obvious, but sometimes you have to do a little investigating to see the extent of what is really going on.

If possible, have a few family members or close family friends visit your parent. This way you can compare what you and everyone else discover. Sometimes close family members overreact from small behavior changes — your parent may need some in-home services as opposed to moving to another home or into long-term care. You may even be in denial, so having someone else observe the situation may give you a more accurate description of how your parent is coping.

Sheila helped open my eyes to how severe the situation was with Mom. I kept saying, "Just give Mom one more year before we rip her from her life." Finally Sheila had to say to me, "She may not have one more year if we don't move her home with us now." Sheila was right and I'm thankful for her honest insight.

1.1 Living conditions

The first sign that your parent is no longer able to cope on his or her own may be the state of his or her home. Your parent may have once been very clean and organized, but now the inside of his or her home is messy and disorganized. There may be dirty dishes piled in the sink or spread around the house, moldy food in the fridge, or no food at all. You may also come across dirty clothes, towels, and bedding. Appliances may be broken or beyond repair or the furnace may no longer work properly or at all. On the extreme side, there could be an infestation of bugs or mice.

Outside the house, the yard may be neglected with signs of many weeds and an overgrown lawn or flower beds. Minor or major maintenance of the home is not being kept up such as broken windows, a leaking roof, or peeling paint. Damaged sidewalks and walkways may cause the person to trip and fall.

Basically, anything around the home that is evidence of poor living conditions is a sign you need to talk to your parent and find out why his or her living conditions have deteriorated.

If the person has a pet, the pet may be malnourished or overfed. In the case of my grandma, she forgot to feed her dog until it was close to death. We had to remove the pet from her home, but the dog had to eventually be put down due to how poorly it was. In Mom's situation, her dogs were grossly overweight from being overfed and not exercised enough.

Another concern with pets is if they are not being kept clean and the elderly person is sleeping with the animals. The bedding may be filthy, the floors unwashed, or there is other animal damage to the home that should have been fixed. Foul odors are another sign due to dirty litter boxes or feces and urine on the floor and stains in the carpet.

1.2 Behavioral signs

Overmedicating can be a common problem with prescription medications as well as self-medicating (i.e., drugs, alcohol, smoking). New habits such as drinking throughout the day or picking up smoking after decades of being smoke-free are all concerns.

The person may be taking a number of medications prescribed by various doctors. Check the labels on your parent's medications for expiration dates and doctor names. If you noticed different doctor names, you need to find out why your parent has been going to so many doctors. Your parent may be forgetting that he or she has seen many different doctors and the medications may be conflicting which is making his or her memory worse. Talk to a pharmacist about the medications your parent is taking; he or she can give you advice and whether or not the medications conflict with each other.

We noticed with Mom that whenever she had a cough, she would take a swig of cough syrup straight from the bottle. We observed her doing this many times throughout the day. She had also begun drinking a bottle of wine every one or two days, which didn't help with her memory or balance. Mom had never been much of a drinker so this came as a big surprise for me. We later discovered the wine was a coping mechanism for her stress.

We also found a newspaper article that Mom had kept saying a daily glass of wine was good for a person, which translated into her telling us a doctor had told her to drink wine every day. We had to wean her from her wine addiction by eventually substituting nonalcoholic wine in the regular wine bottle. Eventually I talked to a pharmacist, with Mom present, about the effects of alcohol mixed with her medication. When the pharmacist explained to Mom that alcohol didn't mix well with her medications, she stopped drinking all together. Hearing this from a professional instead of concerned family members helped her believe the wine was not necessarily good for her in her situation.

If your parent was once a social butterfly, but now he or she refuses to go out, he or she may be socially isolated. You might notice that his or her friends no longer come for visits or he or she no longer makes it to regular social events or clubs. For example, church or some other form of religious contact may have been a staple in your home growing up, but now you may notice your parent is no longer attending services, which could be a sign that all is not right.

Another sign is hoarding. In Mom's situation it was paper hoarding. She kept every scrap of paper she wrote on or notes others gave her for appointments. She did this because she thought it helped with her memory, but instead it confused her because she would refer to old notes and appointment times.

1.3 Physical signs

Has your parent lost or gained a significant amount of weight? In our situation, Mom was extremely skinny, which shocked all of us. She had always been a bit rounder, not overweight, but not skin and bones. We discovered that she no longer had an appetite and if it wasn't for her boyfriend insisting she eat at mealtimes (he was the primary cook in their household), she would have starved herself to death. Chapter 7 goes into more details about problems with eating.

Your parent may be bruised or have cuts or sores he or she can't explain. This may be a sign of falling or may even be a sign of abuse by his or her spouse or significant other. Note that sometimes partners have a hard time dealing with the negative cognitive changes in another person and may no longer know how to deal with the situation. Other partners may have been abusive all along but your parent may have at one time been better at hiding the signs of abuse. Your loved one may show mental signs of abuse by being timid around the person he or she is living with. Maybe he or she cringes when the other person raises his or her voice. (See Chapter 9 for more information about elder abuse.)

The abuse may be the other way as well. As tough as it may be to admit, maybe your parent is abusing his or her partner. Those suffering from the early to mid-stages of AD may inflict violence on those around them because they are confused or frustrated and no longer know how to deal with their emotions.

You may also note that your parent no longer dresses appropriately. For example, he or she may wear pajamas when walking the dog. Or wear a heavy winter jacket when it is the middle of summer or a t-shirt in the middle of a winter storm.

Your parent may be wearing soiled clothing due to incontinence. He or she may not realize that there are stains on his or her clothing or favorite chairs around the house.

Your loved one's driving may be dangerous or erratic. If you discuss this with your parent, you may find he or she becomes defensive or hostile about it. (See Chapter 5 for more information about dealing with driving issues.)

If your parent smokes, you may notice burn marks around the house that weren't there before. You might observe your parent falling asleep with a cigarette in his or her hand while sitting in his or her favorite chair in the living room.

1.4 Financial signs

Bank accounts may be drained with no explanation from your parent as to where the money was spent. Credit cards may be maxed with odd purchases. Junk mail may be piled around the house with requests for donations from legitimate and non-legitimate charities. Mom was giving to every charity known to man, which was depleting her resources slowly and building up the junk mail collection in her filing cabinet.

If there are strange new people in your parent's life who seem to hang around for no reason you can understand, you need to find out who they are and why they are hanging around your parent. There are many people who prey on the elderly with contractor scams, phone scams, and the like. (See Chapter 6 for information about fraud.) If you notice cherished items missing from your parent's home, find out what happened to these items.

You may find bills unpaid or utilities have been turned off due to disregarded or misplaced bills. Or bill collectors have been calling, which can be causing your loved one major stress because he or she doesn't understand why he or she is receiving these calls.

2. Talk to Your Family First

Moving a parent into your home means your life will change. It is a big decision and not one to be taken lightly. You need to discuss it with your spouse and children before you talk to your parent because everyone in your home will be affected.

You should also include your siblings and any other extended family who may have concerns for your parent. Don't force other family members to help if they are not willing or comfortable to do so. It can create resentment, and it may even cause ill-treatment of your parent. Sometimes it is better without family members interfering with their own agendas. The family members that are resistant may get over their resistance in time, but the key is not to pressure anyone. The important thing to remember is that this is about your parent's welfare and not about anyone else's old grudges or unresolved family issues. At this time, past hurts need to be forgiven and everyone needs to move forward for your parent's sake.

2.1 Explaining the situation to your children

This may be a great opportunity for the children to get to know their grandparent; however, you will need to explain the situation to your children about what to expect when Grandma or Grandpa moves in. The Alzheimer Society has some wonderful illustrated children's books that you may be able to borrow from your local organization. By using the children's books, and explaining the disease, it will make it easier for your children to understand when their grandparent has an "off" day.

Your children may need to take on extra chores to help their grandparent. You will want to make sure your children don't resent your parent because of these extra duties. Explain to the children that it not only helps their grandparent, but also helps you and your spouse as well.

Try to make it a positive experience, such as explaining to your children that they are getting older so you are "trusting" them to do more "adult" duties. This may make them feel more responsible and excited to be able to help. It may be as simple as taking Grandma for a walk with the dog every day, or spending time sharing stories with Grandpa while weeding the garden.

You will also need to assess whether or not your parent can stay with small children alone for short or long periods of time. The safety of your children needs to be discussed before the move.

2.2 Talking with your spouse

Consider your spouse's feelings. If your spouse has never gotten along with your parent, maybe moving your parent into your home isn't the best option. Statistics show that many people who take on an ailing relative later get divorced due to the additional stress added to the household.

Will your spouse understand that you won't have as much alone time together? Or that you may not be able to go on dates as often, or family vacations.

You and your spouse need to have a strong connection because there will be hard times and hurt feelings due to the needs of your parent over your spouse's needs. Note that a person with AD picks up on moods better than most people so if there is tension between you and your spouse, your parent will notice. Fighting, yelling, and tension are all much too stressful for a person with AD.

2.3 Consider your relationship with your parent

What about your relationship with your parent? If your relationship has always been rocky, please don't think that it will magically change for the better now. AD can change your parent's personality.

Even if you have always had a wonderful bond with your parent, this may change due to what your parent is going through now. You may find living with your parent brings back bad memories from childhood, which can make you less empathetic to your parent's situation now. Consider talking to a therapist to try to work through the issues so that old problems don't cause friction in your home.

2.4 Work and activity schedules

Do you and your spouse have full-time jobs? If so, consider how you will both manage the caretaking duties while working. You may need to hire someone to come into your home and look after your parent when no family members or friends are available.

In our situation, Sheila and Shawn worked full time, Monday through Friday. I worked at home editing and writing so I was able to move my work to Sheila's home during the week or I would have Mom come to my home. In the evenings I worked at a job outside my home, but my shifts don't begin until either Sheila or Shawn is home from work. We were lucky because of my work schedule, but not everyone works part time or from home.

However, working while around Mom did become stressful because some days she was so agitated I had to get her out of the house to do an activity to decrease her stress. My deadlines, including the one for this book, were long overdue. Luckily, I have some wonderfully understanding clients. Eventually we had to get Mom involved in a day program for seniors so I could stay on top of my freelance work. (See Chapter 8 for more information about adult day programs.)

Depending on how advanced the disease is, you may not be able to leave your parent alone so that means bringing him or her to all family functions, children's sports events, and other family outings. If your family loves camping in the summer, consider how your parent will feel about being in the wilderness. You may need to reduce your camping trips, or find someone to look after your parent while you are away. (Chapter 10 discusses respite care.)

You will also need to consider your parent's activities and medical appointments. When you move your parent, you will spend countless hours setting up medical appointments, filling out insurance forms, changing his or her address on important documents, and traveling to and from appointments. Your parent may also want to be involved with clubs so driving the person to and from his or her activities will take away from you and your family's time.

If you are a part of the "sandwich generation" — supporting your parent *and* your children — you need to schedule yourself some "me" time. If not, caregiver burnout will get you sooner rather than later. (See Chapter 10 for more information about taking care of your needs.)

2.5 Increased living expenses

There may be more household costs depending on whether or not you are going to have your parent contribute to household expenses or not. It is an extra mouth to feed and increased utilities used.

In our situation the heating bills when up drastically because Mom was always cold. We all had to learn to live with a hotter home environment. Even though Mom wore more sweaters, she needed the extra heat. We bought a space heater for her bedroom so she was extra cozy at night.

If your parent insists on paying rent or for some of the food, if he or she can afford it, why not let him or her contribute? This may make the person feel some independence by being able to contribute to the family household expenses. You will need to talk to other concerned family members, such as siblings, about the financial situation. They may not feel comfortable with your parent paying you for any living expenses. Or maybe you are not asking your parent for money to help with household expenses, but you want your siblings to contribute.

Another consideration is increased gas usage in your vehicle. My vehicle's monthly gas expenses doubled due to all the appointments for Mom as well as driving across town many times a week to spend time with her at Sheila's.

Your parent may have special food restrictions due to allergies or ailments so your grocery expenses may increase, especially if you have to buy specific foods for your parent.

2.6 Renovations

Will you need to renovate your home to accommodate your parent's special needs? You may need to add grab bars to the bathtub, wheelchair ramps, or wider doorways for walkers and wheelchairs.

It is important that your parent has his or her own space, a room he or she can retreat to for privacy. In this case, you may need to convert your home office into a bedroom or move one child into another child's bedroom in order for your parent to have a room of his or her own.

If you do need to renovate to accommodate your parent, you may be able to get some tax breaks. Contact your tax authority or tax accountant for more information.

2.7 Create a backup plan

If the living situation doesn't work out, you should have a backup plan in place. For example, one of your siblings will take your parent or maybe even a close friend of the family. You may not realize the extent of how advanced the AD is until the person is living with you, so long-term care may be your only option.

However, give it some time before making any rash decisions. At first, Sheila and I thought Mom was much more advanced in the disease than she was. Once we reduced her stress and she settled in, things were not as bad as they seemed in the first few weeks after she moved.

3. The "Talk" with Your Parent

When it comes time for the discussion to move your parent in with you or another family member, always remember you are changing this person's life at a time when he or she is already experiencing a lot of confusion. Your parent may not realize how much help he or she needs or even why the move is necessary. The person may be in denial or angry because of his or her loss of independence.

You need to make sure the conversation is as positive as possible. In our situation, Mom knew eventually we would come for her because she had to do that for her mother (my grandma). However, it still wasn't an easy topic for Mom to discuss.

Take a moment to imagine your life and how you would feel if someone you knew said right this moment: "You need to move out of your home (and your life) to live with us." You know as of right this moment you don't need looking after; the person with AD may also think that even though it is obvious to you that he or she does need help.

It's scary moving from a familiar situation especially for a person with AD. A person with AD copes with the disease by having routines so that it is easier to remember things. Now this person will have to learn a new routine with your family, and learning may not be so easy at this stage in his or her life.

There are so many mixed emotions to consider when you have the talk with your parent. In our situation it was hard because Mom's boyfriend didn't want to move to Alberta because his family network was in Saskatoon. He didn't want her to move because he felt he needed her there. She felt guilty leaving him, even though she knew it was for the best.

Our conversation included Mom, her boyfriend, Sheila, and I. The four of us sat in Mom's kitchen, where she was most comfortable, and we held her hands as we discussed her moving home with us. We all cried as the conversation progressed. The realization that this would change *all* of our lives was overwhelming.

I felt incredible guilt because I knew how much Mom loved her home, but the proper care wasn't available. We explained this. We also explained that she would need to be driven to and from various doctor appointments. We could help her with the medical jargon and the appropriate steps that need to be taken in the future.

We also explained that one person could no longer be a caretaker because she needed 24-hour care. She was getting lost more frequently while driving or walking to the store. This didn't mean that we had to be shackled to her side all the time. It meant having a presence in the home even if she was in a different room doing her own thing. We stressed that we were not taking away her privacy, but instead we would be there if by chance she felt lost or confused.

Explain to your loved one all the fun things you can do together. In our situation, Mom would have a chance to get to know her grandchildren better. She could go see my nephew, Kaiden, play lacrosse; and my niece, Ashleigh, graduate. Family BBQs; going to church with her son, Shawn; camping; and many other social outings would benefit her socially, which is something that is important for people with AD.

Explain to the person that his or her quality of life will improve. That should be the main reason why you move your elderly parent into your home. Your goal should be to make sure your parent is comfortable and is treated with dignity and respect while he or she is going through this difficult disease.

Tips for your conversation:

- Keep the conversation positive.

- Do not yell or argue because this causes your parent to have stress and with AD, you need to reduce stress.

- Discuss the benefits of moving into your family's home.

- Only make promises you are positive that you can keep. You need to build trust with your parent.

- Include your parent in the planning of the move, but if you notice your parent becoming agitated or stressed during this conversation, break the planning into small tasks so he or she is not overwhelmed.

- If your parent has a house pet, try to accommodate by bringing the animal into your home. Pets are a great comfort (see Chapter 8 for more information about pets).

- Ask for your parent's opinion and incorporate what he or she wants into the planning.

- Reassure the person that you are always going to be there for him or her.

- Do not focus on negative issues or past conflicts. This is about the here and now.

- Focus on the current issues.

- Never talk down to your parent.

Your parent may feel he or she will be a burden to you and your siblings so you need to reassure him or her that he or she will be included as a valued member of your family. You are doing this because you want to help him or her, and to enjoy the time you will have together.

If the conversation isn't going well with your parent, enlist help from others such as doctors or therapists.

3.1 Enlist a doctor's help

Before the move you should talk to your parent's doctor. He or she may be able to help with the discussion about moving in with the family.

We were lucky that Mom's doctor insisted she move home with us. Mom trusted her doctor's opinion so she was more willing to listen to the doctor's advice than to us.

When you are booking an appointment, make sure the medical clerk knows that it is a consult with the family and your parent. The medical clerk may need to book extra time. In our situation, the medical clerk didn't book for extra time (even though I explained the situation), which upset the doctor because it pushed back all of her other patient appointments. In fact, the doctor had us come back during her lunch hour to finish the discussion.

If you feel your parent should no longer drive, talk to the doctor about that as well. Because Mom was moving to a new province, I discussed the situation with my doctor first and he suggested that we have her current doctor remove her license. This prevented her from being mad at her new doctor for taking away a piece of her independence.

Note that many doctors don't like to be involved in the decision about removing a driver's license so you may need to talk to a driver's licensing bureau, which may insist your parent take another driving test to determine whether or not he or she can still drive. (See Chapter 5 for more information about driving.)

Talking with your parent's doctor while your parent is there is a good way to find out about the medical issues that are going on with your loved one. There may be medical issues your parent doesn't understand or has completely forgotten about. You can also get a list of the proper medications and dosages for your parent, which is important.

If your parent has many doctors, then you should take the time to talk with all of them to find out why there are so many doctors treating your parent.

Unfortunately, in many areas, doctors are not taking on new patients so you will need to find a doctor in your area that is willing to have your parent as a patient. I have a wonderful doctor who normally doesn't take on new patients but because I talked to him in advance and said I would like to have the same doctor as Mom, he agreed to have her as a patient. It is beneficial for doctors to treat all the same family members in case there are chronic health problems in the family. It gives the doctor an opportunity to know the family history better and to be able to treat problems within the family.

After you have acquired a doctor in your area for your parent, you will need to contact all the doctors your parent has dealt with in his or her former area. You will need to get all the medical files transferred to the new doctor before your parent even meets the doctor. Depending on how many doctors your parent was seeing, this can be an expensive but necessary endeavor. The cost for file transfers is up to the clinic you are dealing with. As far as I know, there are no regulations or set costs for file transfers. I paid $30 at one clinic because they had to scan all the files into the computer and then transfer them, and it had to be paid by check or cash not debit or credit card. Another clinic didn't charge me at all because it was an electronic-file transfer.

You will need to keep on top of the file transfers because, as in our situation, the scanning of the files was a big task that the medical clerks kept putting off. I had to keep calling to remind them to get it done. I believe it took about three weeks before the files were finally sent. I'm sure they would have never have arrived if I hadn't kept calling.

3.2 Contact a therapist or counselor

If your parent is willing, it may be beneficial to have him or her talk to a therapist or counselor before the move. Your loved one may be going through anxiety, depression, and anger because of the move and from the realization that he or she is losing some independence. A therapist or counselor may be able to help smooth the transition for your parent.

Your parent may want one-on-one time with the therapist or he or she may want to discuss some issues with you there. The therapist may be able to provide some techniques for both you and your parent to deal with the many family issues that can be caused by this major change in lifestyle for all of you.

3.3 Contact the Alzheimer Society

Your local Alzheimer Society or Alzheimer's Association will be able to help you by providing information, brochures, videos, and other helpful tools so contact them as soon as you can. They are the experts and they know the disease having dealt with many people with AD. Tap into that resource because it is free and there for families like yours.

I am so grateful to our local branch because they have been a wealth of information and support for our family.

4. Power of Attorney and Health-Care Directives

As your parent progresses through the disease you will need to take on more responsibility for his or her finances and health care. You will constantly be asked if you have the proper documentation and if it has been "enacted" in order to discuss your parent's situation. Government agencies, medical facilities, credit card companies, insurance agents, and many others will ask for copies of these documents before they will talk to you in regards to your parent.

I discovered using the Power of Attorney and Health Care Directive Mom had certified in Saskatchewan were accepted in some situations, but the wording was different in my province, so many institutions didn't understand exactly what the documents meant. When Mom had signed the documents, they were automatically enacted because that is how they were worded and it was what Mom wanted.

If your parent already has documents in place, but it was certified in a different state or province than the one he or she is moving to, your parent will need to talk to a lawyer in your area. If your parent is too far along in the disease, he or she may not be able to legally sign documents so you will need to talk to a doctor about getting a "doctor declaration" so you can move forward in being your parent's guardian or trustee. You will also need to apply to the local courts so you can be declared as your parent's guardian and/or trustee.

The names for these documents vary depending on your jurisdiction. The financial document is usually called something along the lines of power of attorney, springing power of attorney, or power of attorney for property. The health-care instructions fall under personal directives, medical consents, and health-care directives.

Because there are so many variations in the rules and wording of these types of documents (and I'm not a lawyer), I can't go into the details without writing a whole other book about it. Each area is different so talk to an attorney in your area and find out what steps need to be taken. There are also many good books you can buy or borrow to find out more about this.

The important thing to know is you will need this paperwork in place as soon as possible. You will also need to carry a copy of the documents to appointments, so talk to an attorney right away.

CHAPTER 2
The Memory Book

"Unless we remember we cannot understand."

— E. M. FORSTER

A person with Alzheimer's disease (AD) is prone to mood swings, which can be triggered by a variety of things. The Memory Book has been the most valuable tool for helping Mom to reduce her triggers. Mom's Memory Book and the next chapter's topic of the *Alzheimer's Planner for Caregivers* are the two main reasons I wrote this book.

Mom had been using memory books for at least seven years to keep track of her daily life. It wasn't so much a journal as a reminder of the things she did during the day. It included shopping lists, appointments, conversations, and sometimes she described her feelings or moods if she felt depressed or anxious.

After Mom recovered from her ordeal with the shingles she didn't remember those three weeks at all. In fact, her last memory was her visit in August and it was now October. She had no recollection of Sheila and I traveling back and forth to Saskatoon, and the conversation about moving her to Alberta was gone. But somehow through the sickness she had managed to write sporadic entries into her Memory Book.

The incident that made us realize the value of the Memory Book happened shortly after she recovered from the shingles. I took her to see her best friend for a few days and when I returned to pick her up, she ignored me for the whole half-hour drive home. I thought it was because she may have wanted to stay at her friend's place longer, but when I asked she wouldn't speak to me.

Sheila was away for the weekend so my brother, Shawn, was going to be looking after Mom. I brought Mom home to Shawn's and went to my evening job. I called when I got home from work and asked how Mom was doing. Shawn hesitated before he finally said, "uh, good" so I figured everything was all right. What I didn't know is Mom had picked up another phone and, because of call display, she saw it was me calling. When Shawn was deciding how to answer my question, Mom was glaring at him while holding the phone. As soon as he hung up, Mom began yelling at him saying, "I'm going home to Saskatoon. I'll rent a car if I have to. Tanya is just after my money so I'm cutting her out of my life."

Shawn secretly texted Sheila and asked her to call me and tell me to come over. (I didn't have a cell phone at the time, but after this incident, I signed up for one!) I drove to Shawn's right away. By then, Mom was lying down in her room. I lightly knocked on the door, entered her room, and called her name. She sweetly answered, "Yes" so I asked, "Is everything okay?"

She paused, as I sat down on the bed beside her, her tone went from sweet to pure anger and when she recognized it was me: "NO! EVERYTHING IS NOT OKAY! You want to steal my money. That's why you are keeping me here."

I was a little sorry I sat beside her because I could feel her anger radiating off of her. However, I didn't want to make a sudden move away from the bed in case that made her more hostile so I spoke calmly and asked, "Why do you think I want to steal your money? I haven't asked you for money, and besides I make more in a month than you do so I don't need your money. I never have, and never would steal from you. I know you know this somewhere deep down."

No matter how calmly I talked to Mom, she wouldn't stop yelling at me. Finally she yelled, "GET OUT! GET OUT!" and pointed to the door. I slowly stood up and as I walked to the door I said, "Mom, I know you're having a bad moment but eventually you will come out of it and you will understand that everything is okay." I gently closed the door and joined Shawn in the living room.

We were both in shock. "Is this what we are in store for? Maybe we should send her back to Saskatoon," Shawn said.

"We can't, she'll die there without proper care," I said. "I don't know what to do." To which Shawn said, "I don't know what to do." I think both of us said that phrase over and over again for about 15 minutes because we were totally stumped at how to deal with the situation. I had already begun to notice that Sheila was a calming person to Mom and without Sheila there, both my brother and I were at a loss.

I was about to speak when Shawn motioned for me to be quiet. He had heard Mom open her bedroom door; she stomped down the hallway and into the living room. I had just enough time to say, "Oh Lord, here we go again." I wasn't sure I could handle another tirade after the last one.

She stopped right in front of us and said angrily, "I'm sorry." The words were there, but not the feelings behind them. Both Shawn and I sat in shock because we could clearly see she was still angry but she was struggling not to be.

"I read back a few days in my Memory Book and you are right, Tanya, I know you aren't trying to steal my money. I'm really sorry." She said and then sat down on the couch beside me. She taught us from that moment on, when she is upset about something, we tell her to check her Memory Book. Let me tell you, this book has saved us many times from getting yelled at and prevented her from becoming upset and confused.

The three of us spent the next couple of hours talking about the situation and what may have triggered her mood swing. The reason she was so focused on money is because the week earlier I had gone with her to change her address with the banks and we combined her bank accounts (she had many accounts and she kept thinking she had lost her money, but she had just forgotten which account the bulk of her money was in). We had also done a lot of address changes for her insurance policies and a mail forward. All of this had somehow become jumbled in her mind and because I happened to be the one helping her with the changes, she took out her anger and confusion on me.

I was so glad that I had encouraged her the previous week to write down in her Memory Book every change we made to her bank accounts, address updates, etc. The important thing to note here is she wrote it down as I explained it to her. It was in *her* writing, not mine. If she had seen my writing in her book, I don't think that would have helped defuse the situation because she wouldn't have trusted what I wrote. She trusted herself to write the truth as she understood it.

We also discovered that when I had picked her up from her friend's place that she had thought she was going home to Saskatoon. In the past, whenever she came to visit, she would see the family first and then go to her best friend's house before returning to Saskatoon. With me picking her up and taking her to Lethbridge, it was different from her usual routine of driving herself back to Saskatoon. "Home" was no longer Saskatoon but Lethbridge and this also triggered her bad mood.

She also explained that her mind sometimes gets a "fog" or "cloudy" feeling. At other times she gets so frustrated but she doesn't know why so it makes her extremely angry.

After our long conversation, Shawn said, "You should write everything that happened today in your Memory Book." At first she wanted me to write it down, and both Shawn and I said at the same time, "No way!" I explained how she needed to write it down in her own way so she wouldn't accuse me later of making stuff up and putting it in her Memory Book. We did help her by revisiting the topics so she could remember what happened and how it was resolved.

Later that night, Shawn filled in the evening's events in our family's version of a memory book, the *Alzheimer's Planner for Caregivers* (see Chapter 3). At the end of his notes he wrote: "I love my Mom with all my heart; I wish there was a cure for Alzheimer's."

She went shopping the next day with Shawn and then he brought her to my place for the evening. The first words she said to me were, "I'm surprised you want to see me after yesterday."

I smiled and said, "Oh Mom, it's not the first time you have yelled at me!" This made her laugh because what mom hasn't yelled at her kid at some point in her life?!

1. Introducing the Memory Book to Your Parent

We were lucky because Mom's Memory Book was introduced to us and not the other way around. Your parent may not be the type who enjoys writing, but he or she doesn't have to write pages of prose it can be done in point form, lists, or even sketches if the person likes to draw.

The main use of the Memory Book is to help exercise the mind. It helps keep straight the little things that can't be retained in the mind but instead retained in written form as reminders for the person. In a way, it works as a written form of the short-term memory.

Mom was writing in her Memory Book at one of her appointments with Dr. Derman, so he asked her about it. She explained it to him and he said, "You have inspired me to encourage my other patients with memory issues to create their own memory books."

Many times I've heard others ask her about her Memory Book and comment on what a wonderful tool it is for people with memory issues. Conny Schipper, former Manager of Client Services and Programs, Alzheimer Society of Alberta and Northwest Territories, had this to say about Mom's Memory Book:

"At a recent Alzheimer Café at the Round Street Café in Lethbridge, I sat chatting with Pam, one of our regular attendees, and happened to notice that she was holding a red bound notebook. I commented on the pretty color of the book and asked her if it was a journal. She smiled and told me it was her 'Memory Book,' where each day she records some of the things she has done. She told me that it was a very valuable book for her because she can always look back and see that she has taken a bath on Monday, or gone to an appointment, or did some special thing with a member of her family.

"She told me that she keeps her Memory Book on the coffee table or kitchen table where other members of her family can read it or write in things that have been happening in her life, sometimes adding things that she has forgotten. Pam told me her memory book is a very important communication tool not only for her but for her family members as well.

"I asked Pam and her son [Shawn], who was attending the Café with her, if I could share Pam's Memory Book idea with the other families at the Café and they readily agreed."

To read more about the Alzheimer's Café, see Chapter 8, section 1.

1.1 Finding the right book for your parent

If journaling is new to your parent, you will need to slowly introduce the Memory Book concept. Take your parent to a dollar store and look through the small books to find the right style of book for your parent.

A brightly colored book will be easier to find if it is lost. Also, people suffering from AD usually like bright colors because they are easier to see and the color may encourage your parent to pick it up more often to write in it.

At first we got Mom a bunch of small books that had 50 to 100 pages so it was easier for Mom to carry in her purse. Wherever she went, the book went with her. As her memory became worse and she began to get confused with the dates, we bought her a day planner that had the dates already included with a new date for each page. The problem with a book that has the dates on each page is that some days Mom has more than one page of writing to contribute to the day so if she goes over into the next day, she gets confused with the dates.

Another problem with day planners is that they don't have a large selection of colors to choose from. They are mostly black, which isn't as inspiring. To combat that, you can help your parent cut out pictures and make a collage on the front and back cover of the book. Or, if your parent likes to paint, get some acrylic paints and brushes so he or she can paint the cover.

The more you encourage the person to make the book his or her own, the more inclined he or she will be to use the book.

1.2 What to Include in the Memory Book

The important thing to remember is the book is for your parent so he or she should be encouraged to use it in a way that works for him or her. That being said, you will also need to work with your parent to help remind him or her to write in it.

It is not necessarily a journal, but instead a book of reminders for day-to-day living. Mom's book included shopping lists so every time we went out, she would flip to the last page where she kept her list of things she needed to buy. I learned that I had to get her to cross out the items as she bought them otherwise during our next shopping trip she would want to buy the same things again.

Every morning the day would begin with Mom asking me what day it was (e.g., Monday, November 15, 2012). She would write it at the top of the page and then add what time she got up and had breakfast. Because Mom is never hungry, writing in the book that she ate helped her keep track of meals. Before she started writing in meal times, she would argue with me saying she had already had a meal and sometimes she would refuse to eat.

Another important area was writing that she had a bath and that we did her laundry. I was having trouble getting her to take a bath because she would tell me she had one the night before. Being that I don't live at her house, I would have to text Sheila to ask. Sheila would then tell me that Mom didn't have a bath and by then Mom would be dressed and ready for the day; refusing to take a bath.

As I mentioned earlier, when you are helping your parent with any financial paperwork or changing addresses, encourage your parent to write every step in the book to help remind him or her should any problems arise.

Some other topics to encourage your parent to write about include:

- Family events such as BBQs, grad ceremonies, a grandchild's sports event
- Concerts or movies that your parent attends
- Books your parent is currently reading
- Weather
- Moods and feelings

- Vacations

- Visitors to your home or people your parent visits

- Activities such as going to day programs for seniors

- Going out for dinner or what the person ate that day

- Pictures or news articles

You may also want to glue a map of your neighborhood into the back or front of the book so that if your parent becomes lost, he or she may reference the map in the book. Adding the first name and phone number of the caregiver will also help if the book is lost, or if your parent is lost.

1.3 Making the Memory Book unique

One day I came into the kitchen to discover Mom adding pictures to her Memory Book. The pictures matched the entries so it gave her a visual reminder of something that happened that day. For example, the pure white dog rolling in mud and then coming in the house with a sheepish look. It reminded her of us having to give the dog a bath before Sheila discovered that the family's cute little Shih Tzu was tracking mud everywhere!

Because of digital cameras, getting photos printed right away is an easy task. Even if I only have two or three photos on my camera, every time we go to Walmart, I develop the pictures for Mom so she can add them to a recent entry in her Memory Book. It's not an inconvenience because we are already there shopping and the pictures help Mom to remember recent events.

If your parent has always liked to draw or paint, go to a craft store and get a small sketch book so that he or she can draw or paint. This may be easier for the person to communicate his or her feelings rather than writing a lot of information. A combination of pictures and words can do wonders to help trigger good memories.

1.4 Helping your parent add to the Memory Book

I can't stress enough that important topics such as finances and insurance topics need to be written in your parent's own writing. This way he or she can look back to what was written and trust that it was true as opposed to not recognizing someone else's writing.

Every day before I leave for work, I make sure Mom and I sit down for at least 15 minutes and discuss the day. Whatever Mom hasn't written in the book, I encourage her to add. Mom is fairly good at writing in her book throughout the day, but sometimes we are on the move all day and she doesn't have a chance to write anything so that is when I make absolutely sure I take the time to encourage her to write something about the day. Even if it is only a sentence or two, it helps.

If she, by chance, misses writing in a day she loses that day in her memory. It's like the day never existed so it is important for us, and for her, to make sure that doesn't happen.

If your parent doesn't want to write, don't push your parent to the point of triggering a bad mood. You may have to wait until later in the day when he or she feels more up to writing something.

Mom does leave her book out for the family to read and write in but not every parent may be so trusting of doing this. Leaving her book out, Mom decided this would help her if we could see what she was writing. If we noticed she was having a bad day, we would write words of encouragement and love. My niece, Ashleigh, was good for writing sweet little notes telling her grandma how much she loved her and how she was glad grandma was staying in their home. Mom would pick up the book later and discover the words of love from Ashleigh and giggle and smile.

Having the family write positive notes of love and encouragement can mean a lot to the person with AD. It also can inspire your parent to pick up the book more often in search of notes from loved ones. Even just writing an inspiring quote you've found online can help perk up your parent's mood. Just make sure your parent is comfortable with others writing in his or her book; otherwise, your parent may see it as an invasion of privacy.

However, for the Memory Book to work the best, it is good to have everyone involved and encouraging the person to write in it. At first it may be a struggle, but eventually it can become a part of your parent's everyday routine.

1.5 Take the Memory Book everywhere your parent goes

Mom has a big purse so it was no problem for her to carry it with her wherever we went. However, before we leave the house we always ask, "Mom, do you have your Memory Book?" If she forgot it, she would panic looking for it, so it was up to us to make sure she had the book with her at all times.

Obviously most men don't carry purses or bags every time they go out, and not all women like to haul around a big purse. If this is your situation, you may be the one responsible for carrying the Memory Book whenever you take your parent somewhere. Make it a part of your routine to make sure the book is with your parent wherever he or she travels even if you have to carry it yourself.

2. Help the Person to Manage Triggers

As the AD progresses you may find your loved one becomes easily agitated and can become angry for what *you* believe is no logical reason for it. However, your loved one does have something that is causing him or her to feel stressed. It could be something that happened to him or her days or weeks ago and now the information is just being processed in his or her mind. The person may not even know why he or she is upset. Or, maybe he or she is having a physical problem such as constipation or dehydration or even his or her medication isn't working properly. The important thing is to try to understand what the problem is so you can help the person work through it.

You need to keep calm during a bad episode. If the person is yelling at you, step back slowly and don't yell back. Mom wanted me to make sure I stressed to you readers that yelling at a person with AD is the worst thing anyone can do to him or her. Yelling at a person with AD creates stress and stress makes the memory worse, which leads to more frustration, confusion, and anger.

I worked with Mom to teach her how to do deep breathing exercises such as breathe in slowly through the nose for five seconds then release the breath slowly through the mouth for another five seconds. Whenever Mom feels anxious, we go through the breathing exercise together.

Putting on soothing music or your parent's favorite music may also help distract him or her from the situation. Don't blare the music just have it playing softly in the background. As much as I hate country music, I usually have on the country channel whenever we are at my house or Sheila's because it helps Mom stay calm and relaxed throughout the day. She's always loved her country music!

If possible, during a bad episode, try to change the subject to something more lighthearted. When the person has calmed down, or even a day or two later, you may want to delicately approach the subject again to get to the bottom of the problem so you can prevent another similar episode in the future.

Listening to the person with AD is important to him or her. Mom and I have an open-honesty policy. If she has a bad episode, we don't pretend it didn't happen. We discuss it and try to find out why it happened. During the months since she moved in with us, Mom has built her trust in both Sheila and I and she knows she can talk to us about anything. I cannot stress enough how important it is to listen to your parent, sometimes that is all he or she needs is to be heard.

As mentioned earlier, ask your parent to write in his or her Memory Book because when a bad episode happens, you and your parent can refer to the book to sort out the current confusion. It may also help the person come out of the mood by providing different information to concentrate on such as a happy quote written in the book or a picture that makes him or her smile.

2.1 What causes triggers?

Triggers can be caused by various situations and circumstances. Here's a list of some of the most common triggers:

- Stress

- Fatigue

- Confusion

- Pain or sickness

- Noisy, public areas with crowds or big family events. Big groups can be overwhelming to the person with AD so if you notice your parent becoming uncomfortable, ask him or her if he or she would like to leave or move to a quieter area.

- Yelling or loud noises or loud music.

- Children's toys that have loud sirens or clanking noises.

- Pressuring the person to hurry; for example, you need to get your child to hockey practice on time but your parent isn't moving quickly. Learn to schedule enough time for procrastination and give him or her at least a half-hour warning.

- Making demands on the person. Don't test or push the person for answers because that causes stress and stress causes memory loss, which is frustrating.

- Weather conditions. Gray or windy days are an instant trigger for Mom. She becomes quiet and irritable. Sometimes closing the curtains or using a Litebook helps her feel better.

- Getting lost. Go with the person on walks so he or she doesn't get lost.

- Losing personal items. Help the person find missing items. With Mom she is always misplacing her Memory Book, glasses, and whatever book she is reading. They are usually in one of three places. Get to know the items your parent loses the most and where the items are usually located.

- Trivializing what is going on in the person's life. Don't say, "I understand what you are going through" because you don't. Unless you have Alzheimer's, there is no possible way you could understand exactly what the person is going through. Just listen to what the person has to say.

Try to include the person in planning for special events. I went through a bad episode with Mom one morning about a month before my niece's graduation. Sheila's household was bustling with the topic of grad — grad committees, parties, and the ceremony.

Mom yelled at me one morning saying she wasn't a real grandma (she's a step-grandma to my nieces) and that she wasn't feeling like she had anything meaningful to contribute to the family. When I got to the heart of the matter, I discovered Mom thought she wasn't invited to the grad ceremony because she hadn't had a formal invite. The rest of us just assumed she knew she was going to the grad, which was wrong on our part.

Mom also wanted to shop for a nice dress but she hadn't told me that until this situation came up. I took her shopping right away. It was a lot of fun picking dresses off the racks and having her model them for me and the store clerk. She got her dress and by hanging it in her closet where she could see it every day until grad reminded her that she was a part of the family and that she would be going to the big event.

We have learned to delete the words "remember" and "forget" from our vocabulary when we are talking with Mom. As she explained to us, using the word "remember" such as "remember when we ... " or "don't you remember?" instantly puts her on the spot so even if she does remember, the stress of being put on the spot makes her forget. She feels threatened because then she *can't* remember. It makes her angry and upset. The same goes for asking if she "forgot" about something.

I'm so sensitive to the word "remember" now that when I see a movie or TV show with a character who has Alzheimer's, I cringe when another character asks the person with AD, "Remember, I told you yesterday?"

Ask your parent what he or she feels when you use the word "remember"; you may be surprised how upsetting this one little word can be.

CHAPTER 3

Alzheimer's Planner for Caregivers

"Organizing is what you do before you do something, so that when you do it, it's not all mixed up."

— A. A. Milne

Alzheimer's Planner for Caregivers is a mouthful for the workbook you will need to use constantly while you are taking care of your parent. I needed to give the Planner a name for this book as well as for the worksheets you can order online from Self-Counsel Press. Sheila had named our version of the family's memory book the "Mom Book." However, not all of you readers will be children looking after a parent and not all parents with Alzheimer's are women! So, I apologize for the long name, *Alzheimer's Planner for Caregivers*, and I will mostly refer to it as the Planner throughout the book and this chapter.

The *Alzheimer's Planner for Caregivers* will help you get organized and stay organized during the time you are looking after your loved one. When you realize your parent has Alzheimer's disease (AD) or some form of dementia, things will move quickly. There will be new doctor's introduced into your loved one's life who specialize in different areas of elder care and you'll need to keep track of the new medicines your parent will be taking, what dosage, and what time of day the pills need to be taken.

Note: All the forms at the end of this chapter, along with bonus forms, can be downloaded. See the Introduction chapter for details. At the end of this book you will find a list of all the forms included in the online kit.

1. Building Your Planner

When we first began our journey with Mom, Sheila had a great idea for us to write in a journal to keep the communication open between us, the caregivers. We included notes about doctor visits, financial updates, change of address info, and medications. We eventually began calling it "The Mom Book." We used it constantly to keep track of appointments as well as Mom's moods.

At first we used a thick journal we found in a dollar store, but as the weeks progressed we found it hard to find information quickly because we had to flip back and forth to find crucial information going by our memory of dates.

In this day and age in which everyone likes to type as opposed to write, Sheila found it easier to type her notes and clip them in the pages. However, in the end we decided a binder would hold the information better than a journal-style book.

I bought a binder and filled it with dividers, big envelopes, and pages. It was slightly more bulky to carry to appointments, but the information it contained made life so much easier that size wasn't a concern.

Your first step is to pick up a medium-size binder, preferably one that zips or has Velcro to keep it closed so nothing ever gets misplaced or lost. I found the 1.5-inch NoteTote Binder to be the best for our situation and it was not too expensive.

I also purchased business card holders to put into the Planner for easy access to contact information for doctors, lawyers, and banks.

You may want to label your dividers as follows:

- Behavior or Mood Swings
- Medical Information
- Medicine and Allergies
- Finances and Insurance Policies
- Contact Information and Special Events
- Miscellaneous

The following sections go into more details about what to include in your Planner. Note that the Planner is for you and any other caregivers that are working with your parent. It may be best if your parent doesn't see what is written when it comes to personal notes so as not to upset him or her. You should keep the book private, in order for you to communicate with your co-caregivers honestly or just as a reminder for yourself.

1.1 Behavior and mood swings

Every day Sheila and I type notes about Mom and add it in our Planner. Sheila and I are like two ships passing in the night because when she goes to work, I arrive to start the day with Mom. When Sheila comes home I go to work at my evening job. The Planner has helped us communicate our private thoughts and concerns when it comes to Mom's behaviors and to help prevent triggers. If Mom had a bad night, I will know what to expect the next day from reviewing the Planner.

Some days it is just a line or two saying that it was a good day. It may discuss what we did and what we had for lunch so Sheila knows to make something different for dinner. Other days, the bad ones, we describe as much about the day as possible so that we can figure out why Mom is having a rough day or what may have triggered it.

This section is also handy for doctor's appointments. This way you can describe what has been going on so the doctor can help by looking into medications or maybe there is a medical issue that is causing the problems.

We label our entries with the date and sometimes the time of the events so we can keep track of everything. When Mom goes through what I call "slipping" (i.e., getting worse and not recovering) we document it. Being that the disease progresses, it's good to keep on top of the "slips."

1.2 Medical information

The medical information section of your Planner will be one of the most important areas to keep notes about doctors' appointments and any questions you and your parent may have for the doctors. The medication section is separate; I'll explain why in section **1.3.**

See Samples 1 through 5 at the end of this chapter for what to include in the medical information section.

1.3 Medicine and allergies

Over and over again I was asked by doctors and other medical professionals for a list of the medications Mom was taking. Instead of hauling all the bottles of pills or a makeshift list, I designed Sample 6 which includes the medications, vitamins, and allergies. I added Mom's name at the top of the form and made a few copies to give out to those who needed the information.

You will need to know a lot about your parent's medications, dosages, when the medicine needs to be taken during the day, and if the medication needs to be taken with or without food. You will need to provide this information to doctors, nurses, dentists, optometrists, and so forth. You may even need to provide a copy to an adult day program if your parent is staying for more than a couple of hours a day.

Print a few copies and keep them in your Planner so you have them handy when you go to appointments. If the medical practitioner asks for the information, you will have a copy to give to him or her. This form is also helpful to give to any caretakers or friends and family that may be spending a day or more with your parent.

It's also a good idea to have a weekly pill container that has dividers for breakfast, lunch, supper, and bedtime pills. We also keep a copy of Sample 6 with the bag of prescription refills so we know how to reload the pill container. Keep the container out of reach to prevent your parent from double-dosing.

If you are having trouble with keeping your parents medications organized, you may want to contact the pharmacy to see if it provides a blister packaging service (sometimes called bubble wrap packaging) in which the medications and vitamins are placed in a cardboard sheet with tinfoil backing. It's similar to a weekly pill container in that it divides the medications into the time of day when those pills need to be taken. There is a small fee for this service, and the pharmacy may only want to do blister packs for no more than four weeks at a time.

This section of your Planner should also include information about the medication your parent is taking. Pharmacists can print a copy of the medication information such as the side effects.

With every new prescription Mom gets, I have the pharmacist print the info and then I add it to this section of the Planner. More than once I have had to consult the information because Mom was having a side effect caused by a medication.

At tax time, note that most pharmacies can print a list of all medication costs for the previous year, which you may be able to use for deductions on your parent's taxes.

1.4 Finances and insurance policies

I can't stress enough how important it is to keep your parent's finances separate and organized from your own finances (more about this in Chapter 6). Your parent's money is his or her money, not yours. If you do "borrow" from your parent, note that there could be legal ramifications. Financial abuse is unacceptable (see Chapter 9 for more information about financial abuse).

The financial section of your Planner is not meant to hold all your parent's personal financial details. This is mainly to keep detailed notes about long-term care insurance policies and funding information for seniors in need of government help.

You should have a separate file at home with all of your parent's banking information. You don't want to carry around important financial information that could be comprised if the Planner is accidently lost or misplaced.

This section of the Planner may also include notes about address changes and anything else that affects your parent's finances. You may want to include brochures or pamphlets about tax info that you need to follow up. (See Sample 7.)

In our situation, I constantly had to call and call again to get addresses straightened out. I had to document who I talked to, the date of the conversation, and what was discussed. Be very detailed in your notes because if you ever have a family member who questions your motives when it comes to your parent's finances, having detailed notes will help you explain what you have done and why.

You may also want to keep a folder in this section that includes your expenses (e.g., food, living and moving expenses, clothes, activities) for taking care of your parent. This is the money you have spent that is your own money and not your parent's money. There may be caregiver tax breaks in which you can deduct the expenses for taking care of your parent in your home. Talk to an accountant or your tax authority for more information about caregiver tax incentives.

1.5 Contact information and special events

We had a separate Medical Contact Information form that we kept in our medical section of the Planner (see Sample 2, section **1.2**). You may decide having all contact information in one section works better for you. Design your Planner for what works best in your situation. (See Sample 9.)

We also kept a list of special events such as birthdays and anniversaries so we could remind Mom when the dates are near so she can buy gifts and cards. She was never one to miss a birthday so we make sure to remind her of friends' and family celebrations.

Most people use the calendar provided in their cell phones to add important appointments; however, it is a good idea to have all appointments on a list and hung somewhere in the home so the person with Alzheimer's can see what's upcoming. You never know when your cell can go missing or data could be lost due to some type of malfunction!

Instead of just hanging this form on a wall or the fridge, you may want to instead have a big wall or desk calendar that includes important dates and appointments specifically for your parent. It just depends what works best for you and your parent. A calendar might not provide you with enough space for details, so you may find Sample 8 is handy for the elderly person to access the information quickly and easily.

If you are sharing caretaker duties, having the events in the Planner will help you and your co-caretaker keep organized for events.

1.6 Miscellaneous

You may come up with other ideas for your Planner. Our miscellaneous section was eventually converted to a section entitled "Day Program," which included notes and copies of contracts from the day center Mom began attending as the AD progressed.

You may want to keep important news articles about AD, or brochures you received from the Alzheimer Society in this section.

You should also keep copies of the Power of Attorney, Health-Care Directive, or any other similar legal documents in the Planner. You will be asked over and over again for copies of these forms so that medical professionals, government agencies, and insurance agents can talk to you about your parent's condition. More often than not, most government institutions and medical facilities will not discuss your parent's situation until you have these documents in place so contact a lawyer as soon as possible. You may also need to ask your parent's doctor to enact the forms, but this depends on your jurisdiction.

2. Stay Organized

I can't emphasize enough how important it is for you to stay organized from the day you discuss moving your parent into your home to the time when your parent goes into a long-term care facility. Your *Alzheimer's Planner for Caregivers* will help you stay organized and keep important information together and handy.

You may need to take 15 to 30 minutes at the end of your day to keep your Planner up to date, but it will be well worth it.

You can download the forms mentioned in this book. See the Introduction for details.

Sample 1
DOCTOR'S APPOINTMENT NOTES

Doctor: _____

Your parent may have different doctors for different situations such as the Geriatric Doctor will be the person to talk to about Alzheimer's disease, while the General Practitioner can give advice about every day ailments and injuries.

Leading up to the doctor's appointment, it's a good idea to list the questions or concerns you need addressed by the doctor. Print a copy or save one in a Parent File on your computer and add to it as concerns arise. Take your notes with you to the next appointment and write down the doctor's answers so you have it for reference in the future.

Appointment Date	Question or Concern	Doctor's Advice	Follow-up Information
Example: August 18, 2012 4 p.m.	First visit, what to bring to the appointment?	Medication list and family medical history	Doctor would like to go over the family medical history and review medications.
Example: August 30, 2012	Mom feels anxious lately, what can we do?	Increase anxiety medication and go for more walks on sunny days to relieve the anxiety.	Follow-up appointment in one month, on September 30 to see how the medication and exercise is helping Mom.
Example: September 30, 2012	Mom has a pain in her lower leg.	The start of arthritis.	Also follow up on mom's anxiety and how the increase of meds is working for her.

MEDICAL CONTACTS

Even though the Alzheimer Society is not a "medical contact," they may be able to direct you to doctors or specialists that work with the disease. Plus, the Alzheimer Society is a wealth of information!

Name	Phone Numbers	Address
Local Alzheimer Society (Contact person): *Doreen*	*555-555-4444*	*123 Main Street Open 9-5*
General Practitioner Doctor: *Dr. Joe*	*555-555-5555*	*At the Main Street mall*
Geriatric Specialist: *Dr. Anne*	*555-555-3333*	*#5 456 Main Street*
Other Specialist: *Cardiologist Dr. Tracey*	*555-555-8888*	*8th floor of Hospital*
Optometrist:		
Dentist:		
Psychiatrist or Counselor:		
Pharmacist and/or Pharmacy:		
Other:		

FAMILY MEDICAL HISTORY

All the doctors your parent will talk to will need to know about the family's medical history. This form will help you record the information you will need to provide to the doctors.

Medical Issue	Family Member	Additional Information
Alzheimer's	*Example:* Grandmother	*Example:* Diagnosed in her late 70s
Anxiety		
Asthma		
Cancer		
Depression		
Diabetes		
Emphysema		
High Cholesterol		
High/Low Blood Pressure		
Heart Disease		
Other:		

RECORD OF SURGERIES AND HOSPITAL STAYS

The doctors will need to know the history of your parent's surgeries and hospital stays. Do the best you can to record past events and continue to use this form to document current hospital stays and/or surgeries.

Date	Reason for Surgery and/or Hospital Stay	Doctor	Hospital or Outpatient Clinic
Example: September 10, 2012 to September 15, 2012	Bad fall, bruised ribs	Dr. Drake	General Hospital, Small Town, New York

MEDICAL DEVICES AND SPECIAL NEEDS

You may need to rent, buy, and/or install specialized medical devices for your parent. This list will help you keep organized, especially if you are renting any medical equipment. You can add dates the equipment is due back to the provider and/or when payments are due for the devices. This will also provide you with an easy form to give your parent's doctors, if needed.

Medical Issue	Medical Device and/or Special Needs	Additional Information
Example: Farsightedness	Reading glasses	Only needed for reading
Example: Broken leg	Crutches	Rented from General Hospital Return December 2.
Example: Hearing impaired	Hearing aid	Left ear only
Example: Trouble getting in and out of bathtub	Permanent grab bars	
Example: Trouble walking	Rented walker	Pay $50 every month on the 15th.

MEDICINE AND ALLERGY INFORMATION

Patient: _Bob Smith_

Medications			
Medication Name	**Dose**	**Medical Reason**	**Time of Day and with or without Food**
Example: Aricept	10 mg (1/day)	Alzheimer's	a.m. (with breakfast)
Example: Crestor	20 mg (1/day)	Lower cholesterol	(bedtime)
Example: EpiPen	1 syringe	Allergic to bee stings	Inject in emergencies and then get him to the hospital.

Vitamins		
Name	**Dose**	**Time of Day and with or without Food**
Example: Calcium	(2/day)	(with lunch)
Example: Vitamin D3	(2/day)	a.m./p.m. (with breakfast and with supper)

Allergies
• **Example:** Sulfa • **Example:** Red dye

FINANCIAL UPDATES

Date	Institution	Person Contacted	Phone Number	Details
01/05 /13	RBC	Joan Smith	555-555-2222	Set up online banking
02/08 /13	Insurance Company	Bob Jones	555-555-1111	Set up automatic withdrawal for insurance payments to come out on the 10th of every month.

Date and Time	Event	What to Bring	Additional Notes
Example: *September 2, 2013 7 p.m.*	*Surprise 60th birthday for Mom's best friend, Warren!*	*Potato salad*	*Tom will pick up Mom at 6:30 so she can be there on time.*

Besides keeping a copy of the personal contacts in your Planner, you may want to also keep a copy of this form somewhere that is easy for your parent to find. Keep all the caregiver contact info at the top so that if your parent needs to reach you, your cell number is available at all times for him or her.

Name	Phone Numbers	Address
	Home: Cell:	
	Home: Cell:	
	Home: Cell:	

CHAPTER 4
Adjusting to the New Living Environment

"Reminiscing gives people with Alzheimer's disease control of their situation."

— UNKNOWN

Moving an elderly parent with Alzheimer's disease (AD) can be difficult for the person. A change in the person's surroundings, habits, and routines can be confusing for him or her. There may be nights where your parent wakes up crying because he or she doesn't recognize the room he or she is sleeping in; or he or she may wander looking for familiar surroundings.

It will take time for your parent and your family to adjust to the new living arrangements in your home. Be patient and gently work through the issues as they arise.

1. Helping Your Parent Sort through His or Her Personal Items

How you go about helping your parent decide what to move depends on the amount of personal possessions the person has, and at what stage the Alzheimer's is at. If your parent has a house full of furniture and small items, you will definitely have to reduce the amount of items in order for the person to move into your home. The reduction will also help later on when your parent makes the final transition into a long-term care home.

Talk to your loved one and find out what he or she will not part with. Make a list of the items that will be moving with your parent into your home.

There may be special family heirlooms that your parent would like to give to other family members. Instead of bequeathing the items in his or her will, giving the items to people while he or she is alive may give the items more of a personal memory. If it is a special piece of furniture your parent wants to give to a close friend or family member, your parent may find comfort in visiting that person who has the furniture and enjoying it at the person's home.

It is a good idea to keep a list of who was given what by your parent. Have your parent sign the list when it is completed. This way, if you find down the road that your parent is constantly searching for a specific item that was given away, you can consult the list with your parent. Explain calmly to your parent that he or she gave it away because he or she wanted that person to have the item as a gift. Your parent may feel more inclined to believe you when he or she sees the list and his or her signature at the bottom of it.

If your parent doesn't want to get rid of anything, renting a storage bay or clearing a space in your basement may be the only option at this time. As time passes, your parent may eventually be willing to part with the items he or she no longer needs.

If your parent is a hoarder, you will have your work cut out for you. You may have to clear out the garbage without your parent being there. You may even need to enlist the help of a therapist or counselor in order to find out how to best go about reducing your parent's things.

In our situation, Mom was a bit of a packrat, especially with bits of paper. When I was a kid, paper was expensive so anything that could be written on was saved for notes and lists. I discovered that Mom still hadn't got out of the habit of hoarding envelopes, receipts, and cardboard to write notes on. I had to painstakingly go through each bit of paper making sure I didn't throw out anything that was important.

If you come across old prescriptions, dispose of them. Mom kept ingesting old pills she would come across as she unpacked her boxes. She saw how much that worried Sheila and I, so now if she finds pills she asks us first if she should take them. But that doesn't mean that she won't take any pills she comes across in the future. We keep all pills (i.e., her own and ours) locked away and out of sight.

Another problem was all the clothes Mom had collected over the years. She was a size 4 when she moved in with the family yet she had clothing that ranged from size 6 to 14. There were items that she could no longer wear so I had to remove the oversized clothing when she wasn't around to see me do it; otherwise, she would want to keep everything. I kept the clothing and any other items I removed for about six months until I was positive that she would not ask for any of them — which she never did ask about the missing items.

I also removed torn, damaged, and stained clothing. Mom had a lot of high heels that were chewed up by her dogs. They were unfixable so I threw them in the discard pile. Again, I didn't discard anything for six months to make sure Mom wasn't missing any items she considered important.

If your parent collects figurines, coins, stamps, or anything else, you may need to go through the items and get him or her to pick a handful of favorites while the rest are put into storage or a safety deposit box. If your parent doesn't want to give these types of items away, or sell them, or he or she wants to put them in his or her will, then honor the person's wishes and keep these items safe. Expensive collections such as coins should go into a safety deposit box or safe.

If your parent wants to give you items to be displayed around your home, try to make room for these items. It will make your place feel more like home to your parent, and it will help him or her to feel included in your home life.

Anything that strikes a strong memory for your parent should be kept such as photo albums, letters, or other mementos. Don't bury these away in the closet or storage area because memories are the key to staying connected to your parent. You may find your parent pulls out the albums every now and again to explain the pictures to you or a grandchild. Enjoy those moments. The bonus is you may learn something about your family's history that you never knew before.

After you and your parent have gone through everything, you may need to take your parent to a lawyer to add a codicil of what happened to the items mentioned in the will and that they are no longer available. Items that were given away or sold may have been mentioned in his or her will so it will definitely need to be revised. The last thing you want after your parent dies is to fight with anyone over missing items when your parent was in your care.

Every person's situation will be different but what remains the same is having respect for the person and his or her possessions. He or she has gathered a lifetime's worth of mementos and it's hard to downsize, especially when items have personal meanings that may not be known to you. You may need to take it slow with your parent by taking weeks to sort through the items.

Don't be insensitive when helping your parent sort through his or her items. Don't let your parent see you roughly handling the items or mocking an old sweater that he or she couldn't bear to throw out. Always put yourself in your parent's position and consider how you would feel with others riffling through your personal items.

Your parent is going through a lot of different and confusing emotions so try to make the experience as pleasant as possible. If he or she wants to stop and discuss an item, encourage him or her do so. It may be a way for the person to say good bye to the item. If your parent seems to be agitated or overwhelmed, stop for the day and go for a nice dinner or a walk around the park. As much as you want to get it done and get your parent settled, you need to consider how drastically this situation can affect your parent.

2. Finding Important Paperwork

As I said in the previous section, you may have to sift through a lot of paperwork to find the information you will need. Some of the paperwork to search for includes:

- Birth certificate
- Will
- Power of Attorney, or similar document
- Health-Care Directive, or similar document
- Living will
- Medical history
- Bank account numbers
- Credit card information
- Safety deposit box number and bank location
- Pension documents
- Preplanned funeral documents
- Insurance policies
- Vehicle registration and insurance papers
- Mortgage papers or rental agreements
- Property deeds
- Bills

Depending on how organized your parent is, you may or may not need to hunt for the paperwork. Important documents are sometimes found in the freezer for safe keeping, in between the pages of books, or buried under piles of junk mail. You will need to go through everything to make sure you haven't missed anything important.

3. Preparing Your Home

The room you are preparing for your parent to move into should be made as comfortable as possible. You may want to paint the room to suit your parent's love of bright colors or his or her desire for a neutral tone. If the room was a former nursery, you should definitely update the room from a children's style to a more appropriate style for your parent. The goal is to make your parent feel at home in your home. If he or she is waking up to a mobile hanging from the ceiling, that will not add to the comfort level of your parent.

Enlist your parent's help on deciding what colors to paint the room and what curtains or blinds to add. You may want to shop for new furniture that will fit the room better than the furniture your parent currently owns. For example, the new room may be small and will only fit a double or single bed as opposed to a queen- or king-sized bed. Maybe a smaller bed will mean more room for storage such as dressers, chests, and a desk. Don't push your parent to buy new or used furniture if he or she wants to keep his or her current furniture. Your parent's furniture is familiar so it may bring comfort having it in his or her new room.

Mom didn't have a lot of furniture that she wanted to bring with her. Actually, the only furniture she did want to keep was a chest that is older than I am. Sheila already had a bed and dresser, and Mom was thrilled with the new desk and bookshelf we bought her as moving-in gifts. She was fine with the change of furniture, but not everyone is like her.

3.1 Physical disabilities

You may need to prepare your home by doing some renovations. Note that you may be able to get tax deductions from caregiving expenses for altering your home to accommodate your parent. Call your accountant or tax authority to find out more. If you are entitled to benefits, make sure you save all the receipts for tax time.

If your parent is in a wheelchair, you may need to add ramps and widen doorways. Or if your parent has trouble with mobility, you may need to add railings along the walls, and grab bars in the tub and around the toilet as well as adding a nonslip mat to the bottom of the tub.

Find out what your parent needs before you move him or her into your home. Consult with your parent's doctor as well as home health-care stores, which have many elder care supplies available.

3.2 Make your home safe

You won't know the extent of your parent's Alzheimer's until you live with him or her. We assumed Mom was safe to wash dishes; however, we caught her using a poisonous cleaning agent instead of dish soap so we knew we had to make some adjustments. The dish soap was put in a spot Mom could see as soon as she turned on the water. The cleaning agents were pushed far under the sink and behind harmless items such as garbage bags.

If your parent is more advanced in the disease, you may need to add child-proof locks to some of your cupboards to prevent your parent from cooking with or using something dangerous (i.e., knives, cleaning products).

I learned at a meeting about Alzheimer's patients that they don't always feel hot or cold. For example, scalding hot water may not register to a person with AD. You may need to turn down the temperature of your water heater or install an anti-scalding device, also called Temperature Activated Flow Reducer (TAFR). These are easy to install, and their purpose is to stop water flow when the temperature gets too hot.

If necessary, you may need to purchase electrical outlet covers to prevent your parent from getting electrocuted. Or you may need to get devices with timers such as space heaters that shut off after a certain amount of time.

When Mom came to visit me years ago (this was when she was first showing signs of AD), she just about burned down my apartment because she left her curling iron on and touching the wall. When she moved in with Sheila, we decided it would be a good idea to get rid of the curling irons. Instead, Mom goes for regular perms. She likes to get dolled up every six weeks or so with her regular hair appointment and we breathe a sigh of relief because Sheila's house won't burn down due to a curling iron left on! Work with the disease and how it changes your parent. In most situations you should be able to figure out a reasonable solution for everyone.

If you don't want your parent to cook, you may have to find a way to keep the stove from being turned on. You can remove the buttons that turn on the burners. You can also purchase a stove monitor that automatically shuts off the stove if someone hasn't been in the kitchen for 5, 10, or 15 minutes. There are also newer stoves on the market that include a lock-out feature where it locks the oven doors and disables the controls. Or it may be as simple as attaching a note to the stove as a reminder that your parent is "retired" from cooking, which he or she may find funny and he or she may enjoy not having to cook anymore.

In our situation, Mom loves that Sheila is a great cook and appreciates that Sheila doesn't ask her to help with dinner preparation. Mom has never liked to cook, but she'll happily do dishes!

As the disease progresses, a person with AD is more prone to slips and falls. Remove scatter rugs and rugs that are frayed. Also consider adding pictures or decals to patio doors so that your parent doesn't walk into the glass doors. Sharp edges on furniture and glass tables can also be cause for concern if your parent is having mobility issues.

Reduce clutter or excess furniture in your home. As the disease progresses, you may notice your parent's motor skills are not as good as they used to be so removing excess items can help prevent your parent from bumping into things or tripping and falling.

Cords were a problem when Mom moved in. If there was an extension cord attached to a TV, computer, or other electrical device, she didn't see them and would constantly trip over them, which yanked the devices to the floor. It's not that she has bad eyesight; she just doesn't notice cords anymore. We rearranged appliances and gadgets so no cords were anywhere she could trip. That was no easy change since everything is electronic these days!

Increasing light in each room will not only help brighten the person's mood but also reduce shadows. Some people with AD find shadows very scary. At night, you may need to add a night-light to the bathroom and hallway so your parent knows to follow the light to the bathroom. You may even find that leaving the bathroom light on is helpful for your loved one.

If your parent will be left alone for short periods of time, you may want to consider investing in a special service such as Lifeline, which is a Medical Alert service. Your parent can wear a pendant or wrist-style Help Button, which he or she can push for help. It also provides a Lifeline with AutoAlert services, which places a call if your parent can't push the button but a fall is detected by the device. There are also services such as TeleCare which can monitor stove and home temperatures as well as detect falls and even floods in the home.

3.3 Be prepared for wandering

When mom would come over to my place shortly after she moved, she would try to wander. I would often catch her sneaking out the side door. The problem was she was in an unfamiliar area so if she walked around the block on her own, she kept circling the block because she couldn't recognize my home. My husband, Darren, stopped her one day and asked if she wanted to come in the house. She looked at him curiously, and then she recognized him and walked into the house. He told me later that he believed she would have kept on walking if he hadn't said something.

After that, I would go for walks with her and the dog and we would take the same path. The more familiar she is with the area the more chance that if she does wander it will be along the same route we normally take. It also gives me a starting place of where to look for her if she goes missing.

No matter how much you try and prevent bad things from happening they can and do happen, so it's better to try to work with the disease and take precautions. My friend, Janet Cook, suggested that I also point out a gas station or business along the route in case Mom gets lost in the winter. "This way she may be more inclined to enter the business than to keep wandering around out in the cold."

To prevent wandering, especially at night, you may want to add a Confounding Door Lock to your front and back doors. It doesn't look like a lock and it has a trick to opening it that people with AD have trouble figuring out. The Confounding Door Lock should either be put high or low on the door so that your parent doesn't consider it a lock.

You may want to consider setting up an alarm system so if a door opens in the night or day when it shouldn't you will know your loved one may be in a wandering mood. Even just hanging bells above the doors will alert you to anyone coming or going.

Sign up your parent for the Alzheimer Society Safely Home® program. There is a one-time fee ($35 at the time of this book's printing), and your parent will receive an identification bracelet and identification cards. If your parent becomes lost, the person who finds your parent can look at the bracelet for your parent's name and ID number. It also tells the person to call the police, and the police will use a special database to find your parent's address and emergency contact person.

Keep a recent photo of your parent handy just in case you need to show it to others when you are searching for your parent.

If you know your neighbors, introduce your parent to them. Return to your neighbors at another time without your parent and ask your neighbors to let you know immediately if they see your parent wandering alone. Explain that your parent has Alzheimer's and you are trying to set up preventative measures to protect your parent from getting lost.

You will constantly walk a very fine line of what your parent may see as you keeping him or her as a prisoner, and how you see it as keeping him or her safe. If your parent is feeling trapped, maybe you need to take him or her out more or get him or her into some social programs (see Chapter 8 for more informtion about day programs).

3.4 Making adjustments and incorporating house rules

Many times you will have to adapt your way of living to the way of your parent because it will help prevent triggers. However, there are some house rules that you will not be able to bend for your parent such as bed-times for your young children or overfeeding the dog or cat.

Sheila had to learn to relinquish some control of her kitchen. At first it was annoying because she could no longer find anything when she was cooking, but now Sheila jokes about the daily "Easter egg hunt" for dishes! Mom elected herself the household dishwasher even though Sheila has a perfectly good dishwashing machine! Having a job in the house makes Mom feel like she is contributing and it retains some of her independence.

For the house rules that you cannot change to accommodate your parent, you will need to explain why you have the rules and how you can work together to make the rules work. For example, Mom overfed her dogs in Saskatoon. Sheila's family dog, Amy, is a dog that does not eat human food so she doesn't beg at the table. This was a challenge for us to get Mom not to sneak food to Amy. We worked with Mom by letting her give Amy one dog treat — just one — after dinner. This became a habit for Mom and she stopped feeding the dog scraps from the table. Every now and again we have to remind her not to give Amy more than one treat, we use small suggestions and we never get angry at her for doing it.

4. Dealing with Elderly Addictions

Prescription drug abuse among the elderly is a growing problem due to double-doctoring (going to multiple doctors for various or duplicate pre-scriptions). As I have said throughout this book, go through your par-ent's medications, talk to his or her doctor, and find out what your parent should be taking. If your parent is addicted to painkillers or sleeping pills, talk to the doctor about how to help your parent withdraw from the medications. It may be that double-dosing is causing more memory loss than necessary for your parent.

If your parent has a long-time addiction to alcohol or illegal drugs, you will need to talk to a doctor about what to do. Each situation is differ-ent so withdrawal may need to be done with medical supervision.

The antismoking campaign has almost won its battle with rising cigarette costs and the banning of it in most places in North America. More times than not, young families don't allow smoking in their homes so what do you do if your parent smokes and your home is smoke-free? Do you allow your loved one to smoke in your home or the garage or an unused porch? You may be able to convince your parent to try quitting by using electronic cigarettes, which may be a good substation if your parent is used to having a cigarette in his or her hand. There are also nicotine patches and inhalers. If your parent is having a hard time quitting, talk to the doctor and see if he or she can give your parent some advice. There are also many good government antismoking programs that can help your parent quit.

If you can't get your loved one to quit, you may want to purchase The Smoker's Apron. This apron protects your parent from burning his or her clothes and his or her body.

5. Create Jobs in the Home

Jobs or chores may be important to your parent so he or she can feel productive. If he or she wants to help around the house, assess your parent's strength and endurance. Make it so the tasks are small but fulfilling.

One day, early in the fall, Mom came outside to help me rake the leaves. I have a huge yard with 19 trees. I discovered that once Mom started raking she wouldn't stop until we were finished. She wouldn't stop for water or to sit down until I finally convinced her we could work on it another day. After that, if I was working in the yard, I would give her small tasks such as weeding the small strawberry patch or setting out the sprinklers.

Make sure the chores are light in duty and not something the person can get hurt doing. Some simple but helpful tasks may include:

- Folding laundry
- Washing dishes
- Dusting
- Sweeping
- Mopping
- Vacuuming

Letting your parent accomplish small tasks independently can give him or her a sense of purpose and a good feeling about contributing to the household.

Sheila went through guilt about letting Mom do any cleaning. She wanted to treat Mom like a guest; however, Mom was no longer a guest but a member of the household. When Sheila was finally able to rationalize this, she felt better about Mom doing chores around the house.

Also, be sure to thank your parent for a job well done *every* time he or she does something around the house. You may remember that you thanked him or her the last time and the time before that, but your parent might not remember. So always acknowledge his or her help.

If your parent doesn't want to do a job, don't force him or her to do it. He or she may or may not in time ask for duties. Let it be your parent's decision.

6. Include Humor and Love into Your Daily Lives

On our first visit to see the General Practitioner Mom was in a foul mood. She wouldn't tell me why until halfway to the appointment when she began yelling at me.

"I'M A HOSTAGE! YOU'RE KEEPING ME PRISONER!" She roared. I was in the middle of driving on a busy road with no place to stop. I was scared she was going to jump out of the car but I didn't want to hit the lock button because then that would prove to her she was a prisoner. (As a side note, if you feel your parent may try to jump from a moving vehicle, you may want to turn on the child locks so this doesn't happen. It's better to be safe than sorry.)

This happened around the time she was beginning to come out of the shingles and delirium from the infection. We didn't know yet that she couldn't remember agreeing to move to Alberta so I had no idea why she was screaming at me. I tried to calmly explain I was just taking her to the doctor to introduce her to him. She quieted down and sat in her seat with an angry expression.

Thankfully we made it to the doctor's office without her jumping from the car. I slipped a note to the medical clerk explaining Mom had Alzheimer's and that today was a bad day for her moods. I also added that the clerk might want to warn the doctor.

The clerk handled the situation professionally and quietly. The doctor was prepared when he came in the room and introduced himself. He talked to her like a friend, which helped put her at ease. The doctor's calm demeanor seemed to help perk up Mom and her tension seemed to release. It was basically an introduction to the doctor to begin the process of getting her a proper diagnosis for Alzheimer's. The first meeting was nonthreatening so Mom immediately decided she liked the doctor! I'm so thankful to Dr. Derman for how he treated her with compassion and empathy.

I texted Sheila before we left the doctor's office and asked that she be at home when we got there. I had to go to work and I didn't want to leave her with my teenage niece in case she began yelling at her. Mom was silent and had returned to being angry at me on the drive home.

My nose had been itching for the past hour and when I finally looked in my rearview mirror, I was embarrassed to discover what had been causing the itch.

"Thanks Mom for telling me I had a booger hanging out of my nose the whole time we were at the doctor's!" I figured if anything would get her to laugh, that would.

She finally looked at me and then at my nose (and the booger) — she burst into laughter! For the rest of the way home she couldn't stop giggling. When we walked in the door, Sheila greeted us expecting the worst. She asked apprehensively, How was your day, Mom?

"It was fantastic!" She said, and she meant it. Sheila's eyes widened in surprise as did mine, but just a simple funny comment kicked her out of her bad mood.

Humor is so important when dealing with Alzheimer's disease. Mom has a wicked sense of humor and gets us every now and again with a good joke or story. For me, a stupidly embarrassing booger managed to help snap Mom out of a bad mood that had lasted hours. Use whatever works because you may be surprised at the response.

We also give Mom lots of hugs and we tell her often how much we love her and appreciate having her here with us. She needs positive affirmation and we gladly give it to her. When she is having a bad day, I hug her often which helps bring a smile to her face. If your parent accepts hugs, give him or her hugs and do it often.

CHAPTER 5

Who to Contact about the Move

"As of 2012, there were 7,356 allopathic and osteopathic certified geriatricians in the US — one geriatrician for every 2,551 Americans 75 or older. Due to the projected increase in the number of older Americans, this ratio is expected to drop to one geriatrician for every 3,798 older Americans in 2030."

— AMERICAN GERIATRICS SOCIETY
GERIATRICS WORKFORCE POLICY STUDIES CENTER (GWPS)

Be prepared to spend a lot of time on the phone after your parent's move. You'll need many copies of the enacted Power of Attorney (or equivalent) and Health-Care Directive (or equivalent) to mail or fax to government agencies, health professionals, and financial institutions in order to talk to them about your parent's situation.

You will find yourself calling the same places over and over again to make corrections and updates. In our situation, Mom moved from an address that was similar in house numerals to my address (e.g., former address 2225, new address 225). A strange coincidence that caused endless problems of having to call places and correct the address because the old house number kept being used because it was so similar to the new address!

If you are sharing caretaker duties with another family member, discuss which home the mail should be sent to. Since I was taking care of the finances, Sheila and I decided it would be best if I received Mom's mail.

At Christmas time, when Mom filled out her Christmas cards, I made sure she wrote Sheila's address as the return address so that if Mom's friends wanted to send her personal mail, it would come directly to her. This way no important information is delivered to Sheila's that can get lost or misplaced by Mom, which reduces her stress and mine! However, it makes her happy to receive a card or letter in the mailbox at her home.

1. Who to Contact

You will need to document everything when you are changing over addresses and updating accounts. Have your *Alzheimer Planner for Caregivers* handy every time you make a call. These are some of the detailed notes you will need to record:

- Person's name whom you talked with

- Phone number and extension number

- Name of the company

- Date and time of call

- What date to follow up

- What was discussed (make sure you write this in as much detail as possible)

You may want to have a list of questions ready before you make the call. For the first while, until all the places have the Power of Attorney, you may need your parent beside you so he or she can give the company permission to talk to you.

When calling, you will also need to provide a lot of personal information about your parent. Depending on who you are calling, you may need the following information:

- Your parent's birth date (day, month, and year)

- Last address

- New address

- Full name

- Health-care number

- Social Security Number or Social Insurance Number

- Details of why you are calling

The following sections discuss in detail what steps you should take and who you should contact.

1.1 Mail forward

The first step you should make is going to your local post office to set up a mail forward. The post office usually gives you the option of a 3-, 6-, or 12-month mail forward service. Sign up for the 12-month option. The reason for this is you may not know for sure if your parent has yearly bills coming in, so along with regular monthly bills, you need to make sure you don't miss any insurance payments or other bills due throughout the year.

After the first year had passed, I asked the post office to extend the forward for one more year just in case I had missed anything. Sure enough, I had missed contacting one business my mom dealt with on a yearly basis.

1.2 Health care

If your parent has state or provincial health care, you will need to contact the former jurisdiction as well as the new jurisdiction. Besides the mail forward, setting up your parent's health care should be first on your list of things to do.

I had set up Mom for health care in Alberta, which I thought would automatically cancel her health care in Saskatchewan. It didn't. As the Saskatchewan representative explained to me, "Sometimes the new province will contact the old province of residence, while other times no contact is made."

If your parent is covered by the United States Medicare system, it is very important that you contact both the old jurisdiction and new jurisdiction so your parent doesn't lose any benefits he or she has.

Contrary to popular belief about the Canadian health-care system, not all services are free, especially when moving your parent from province to province. The two things that are covered by Canadian health care are hospital stays and doctor appointments. Ambulance services, medications, and so forth are not covered unless the person has an exceptional health-care insurance plan.

For example, if your parent needs to have a bone density test for osteoporosis or any other special care when moving him or her to a difference province, contact the old province's health care and ask if it will cover the cost. If not, wait until the new health care begins for anything that is not an emergency.

In Canada, it can take three months from the date of the move before the new province of residence will send a new health-care number and provide services. When we moved Mom, she was suffering from a bad case of shingles so she needed constant medical attention for three weeks. Some services weren't available such as Home Care because it wasn't covered by her former province with her now living outside of that province. Some of her medications weren't covered either, but we saved the receipts because they were tax deductible.

I had to apply for a new birth certificate for Mom before I could get the health care set up. Mom only had a copy of the original long version birth certificate, which the registry office would not accept because it didn't have a registration number.

1.3 Birth certificate

If your parent doesn't have a birth certificate, it's a good idea to apply for one just in case you need it when updating your parent's files. As I mentioned in the previous section, I couldn't get Alberta health care until I had a proper birth certificate.

Mom was born in eastern Canada, so I had to contact that province's registry and then it took eight weeks before we received the birth certificates. I ordered both the long and short versions of the birth certificate just in case either one was needed. So far, I've only need the short version but who knows if someone will ask me for the long form someday. At least I've got it, if I need it.

1.4 Banks

Chapter 6 goes into more details about finances, but I wanted to address it here as well. In Mom's situation, she had many bank accounts from different banks. This made it extremely difficult for her to keep track of her finances.

I organized her banking into two accounts — one for her bills and savings and the other for spending money. I set up all her payments to automatically come out of one account so I could keep track of what was being paid. This made Mom's life so much easier and less complicated.

Each month I would print out her bank statements and she would go through all her debit receipts checking off her purchases and then stapling the receipts to the bank statements. This is something that she had done ever since I can remember. As the disease progressed, she eventually asked me to take over this task. So every month I go through the information with her so she is still part of the process.

We also set up the accounts so that we are joint parties. This way, if I have any questions, I don't have to bring in the Power of Attorney every time I go to the bank.

Any banking I do for Mom, I talk to her about it first and I get her to record the conversation in her Memory Book. Even though she may not remember the conversation, I know I've got her opinion first before I make updates. With her recording it in her Memory Book, she has a record of the discussion in case she has any questions for me later. I also record the information in the *Alzheimer Planner for Caregivers* so that I remember what I did and why.

1.5 Insurance companies

I found insurance companies the most tedious to deal with. It took multiple phone calls and talking to various agents, mailing letters, and so forth the get all the information I needed to know.

Mom kept some insurance files up to date while others I had to search for to make sure we got all of them updated. Some insurance payments were made by check while others were paid through automatic withdrawal through her bank and through various accounts. I set up all the insurance policy payments to be withdrawn from one account. I also made sure I had the most current copies of the policies for reference.

The problem with insurance companies is that they seem to always be changing their names, brands, and so forth. One insurance company will get taken over by another, and then another bigger insurance company will take over that company! Mom had a lot of paperwork for what seemed like different companies, but instead it was the same policy that had been passed through different insurance company takeovers. It took me awhile to straighten out all of the policies.

Some policies may need to be canceled. She had a safe driver policy that was no longer necessary because she was no longer driving. Even after I canceled it, they kept charging her the monthly fees, so I had to keep contacting the company to cancel it and ask that the company refund the fees charged after the original cancellation date.

1.6 Pensions

If your parent has a pension plan, you will need to contact the pension provider to update his or her information. Again, you will need to send the provider a copy of the Power of Attorney before a representative will help you with the address update or give you any information about the pension.

In Canada, you will need to call Service Canada to make changes to your parent's Canada Pension Plan (CPP), Old Age Security (OAS), and Guaranteed Income Supplement (GIS). Also, if your parent has a private pension from a former employer, you will need to contact that company's human resources department to update your parent's account.

1.7 Tax authority

Don't wait until tax time to contact the tax authorities. Your parent may be making quarterly tax payments or receiving some kind of tax payback, so it is important his or her tax authority is up to date on your parent's current address and bank account (if necessary).

In the US, call the Internal Revenue Service (IRS), and in Canada, call the Canada Revenue Agency (CRA). You may need to send a copy of the Power of Attorney so if you have any tax questions, a representative can help you when it comes to your parent's taxes.

1.8 Closing accounts

Since your parent is moving, you will need to contact companies such as the following to close accounts:

- Gas company

- Electrical company

- Water company

- Phone provider (both home and cell phone providers)

- Cable or satellite provider

- Internet services (this may mean setting up a new email address for your parent so make sure you help your parent contact everyone who emails him or her at the old email address)

- The city for any property taxes or other city billings such as garbage, recycling, etc.

- Put a stop on newspapers, and a forward for magazines and any other newsletters

If your parent is leaving a significant other or roommate, the bills may need to be transferred to his or her name. This may be something that you need to work with your parent's partner or roommate to get this done.

It is very important that your parent's name comes off shared bills because if anything fraudulent happens, or if the former spouse or roommate stops paying the bills, your parent can be liable for those debts.

1.9 MedicAlert and Safely Home®

If your parent has life-threatening allergies, contact MedicAlert and sign up for its services. This could save your parent's life. If your parent is registered with MedicAlert, make sure you update his or her address and also make sure every time medications are changed you tell MedicAlert.

As mentioned in Chapter 4, section **3.3**, the Alzheimer Society provides a program called Safely Home. Once you pay the one-time fee, your parent will receive a bracelet with his or her name on it, and a phone number on the back of it to call if a stranger finds your parent lost or confused.

1.10 Preplanned funeral policy

If your parent has a preplanned funeral policy, make sure you contact the provider to find out the details about the plan. Mom's plan was easily transferred to her new province, but some services aren't available in the new jurisdiction.

1.11 Friends and family

You may need to help your parent contact friends and family about the move. Some friends your parent may only keep in contact with once or twice a year by mail, so it is important to go through your parent's address book and find out who your parent would like to still keep in touch with.

Buy a nice package of blank cards and encourage your parent to write his or her contacts a note explaining that he or she is moving. Remind your parent to add his or her new address.

2. When Your Parent Owns His or Her Home

If your parent owns his or her home, you will need to have a family discussion with your parent and all concerned family members about what to do with the home. If everyone is in agreement, you may decide to sell the home. Talk to a lawyer who specializes in Elder Law and who can give you more advice about selling your parent's home.

If you are going to sell your parent's home, you will need to contact the bank that holds the mortgage, a realtor, maybe a home inspector, and a lawyer who specializes in real estate.

Note that it is usually easier on a senior if he or she packs up and moves out of the home before the for sale sign goes up. However, most insurance companies don't want to insure an empty home (i.e., no one is currently residing in the home).

Contact your parent's home insurance agent and discuss the situation to find out how to keep the home insured while it is on the market. Remember to cancel the insurance when the home is sold.

In the US, you can contact the National Association of Senior Move Managers (NASMM), which provides "innovative programs and expertise related to senior move management, transition, and relocation issues affecting older adults."

If your parent's home was the family home you grew up in, be prepared for your own emotions as well as your parent's when letting go of this place filled with family memories. Be sensitive to your parent's emotions because this was a place that meant a lot to him or her.

3. Health-Care Providers

As mentioned in Chapter 1, you will need to gather all of your parent's medical records and have them forwarded to his or her new doctor. This can be expensive because file transfer costs are usually up to the discretion of the clinic and each clinic will charge different fees. You may need to continually call the clinics to make sure the files are transferred *before* your parent's first visit to the new doctor.

You will also need to contact any specialists your parent dealt with so that the new doctor can have a full picture of your parent's health. For example, if your parent was seeing a cardiologist, then you will need to make sure those files are forwarded.

You will need to contact former dentists, denturists, hearing specialists, optometrists, and psychiatrists as well. Once your parent is settled, you should set up appointments with new dentists, optometrists, etc. in order to make sure your parent has no dental issues, his or her glasses are the correct prescription, etc.

When Mom recovered from her shingles, I set up an appointment to have her teeth checked and cleaned because Mom couldn't remember the last time she was at a dentist. I also took her to the optometrist and we discovered her current prescription was too strong, which was causing her eyes to become sore.

Our General Practitioner also referred Mom to get a bone-density test because as women get older, osteoporosis can be a concern. He also got Mom into a Geriatric Specialist so that we could get Mom started on the Alzheimer medications.

Basically, you want a full medical evaluation of your parent so you know how to care for him or her properly. You will need to set up breast examines or prostate exams for cancer screening. Taking preventative measures is better than having a serious health issue suddenly arise. The General Practitioner will also appreciate having all your parent's medical information so that he or she can properly care for your parent.

4. Asking Your Parent to Relinquish His or Her Driver's License

It's never easy for a person to relinquish his or her driver's license. Having a driver's license is a form of independence, freedom, and mobility so when it is taken away, your parent may become extremely upset. Alzheimer's disease can rob a person of his or her ability to drive as well as his or her insight that his or her driving is now impaired and dangerous.

Unfortunately, unless your parent is willing to relinquish his or her driver's license, you may have to enlist the help of a doctor or the Motor Vehicle Department. Currently there is no North American standardized testing to determine whether or not a person with AD can safely drive a vehicle.

AD can affect the person's judgment, visual perception, and physical coordination. Signs that your parent may no longer have the ability to drive include:

- Increased traffic violations

- Accidents whether minor fender benders or more serious

- Trouble understanding road signs or getting confused at traffic lights

- Getting lost (e.g., when driving a normal route, forgetting where to turn)

- Misunderstanding directions

- Visible agitation and nervousness when driving

- Excessive speeding or going too slow causing danger to others on the road

Mom was upset to lose her license even though driving was a very stressful activity for her to do in her later years. She was also extremely dangerous on the road and we feared if she didn't kill herself, someone else would be hurt or killed.

I talked to my doctor before the move and he suggested talking to her former doctor and having that doctor send in a letter to the driving authority to help get the process started of canceling Mom's license. This way, if Mom was extremely upset about it, she would be mad at the old doctor instead of the new doctor; this would prevent harm to the new doctor's relationship with Mom.

We didn't have to get a doctor to help us encourage Mom to give up her license. She agreed after I explained to her that we would drive her wherever she needed to go. Mom found after awhile that she enjoyed being a passenger because she could look at houses and people walking on the street instead of concentrating on driving. This reduced her stress immensely.

You may find your parent is willing to listen to a doctor about the effects of Alzheimer's on driving. You could ask the doctor to write on a prescription "Do not drive," this way it is on a professional looking piece of paper that your parent can refer to if the topic of driving comes up again. It can be pasted into his or her Memory Book as well.

You may have to write a letter to your local motor vehicle licensing bureau explaining your parent's situation. Include your parent's full name, date of birth, addresses (old and new), and driver's license number. The driver's licensing bureau may ask the person to come in for a road test. In many jurisdictions, driver's licensing bureaus are beginning to request elder people of a certain age to retest yearly so this may not come as a surprise to your parent. The bureau will keep your letter confidential in most cases.

If you don't always have time to drive your parent to and from places, you may be able to find driving services that are available for seniors in your area. Note that as the disease progresses your parent will not be able to take public transit such as buses because he or she may become confused and not know what stop to get on or off at.

If your parent owns a vehicle, you may need to sell it. Also, you will need to cancel the vehicle registration and insurance.

Your parent will still need picture identification, which your state or provincial registry should have some form of government picture ID that your parent can apply for. He or she can also use an updated passport if he or she has one.

Note: If your parent still insists on driving even after his or her license is taken away, you may have cause for concern that he or she will steal your vehicle's keys and drive away. Reduce this risk by hiding the keys. Also, do not leave your parent in a running vehicle even if it is just for a quick second to go in the house or a store to get something.

5. Living Will

Your parent will need some form of living will. Each state and province, and even each city has different names and documents for living wills. For simplicity's sake, I'm going use the name, living will.

A living will is different from a last will and testament (i.e., instructions on what to do with the person's belongings *after* he or she dies). A living will provides family members and medical personnel with written instructions about the level of care and medical treatment your parent wants in the event he or she is unable to express his or her wishes verbally during an emergency. A living will can be modified anytime during your parent's life as circumstances change.

In my area, the long-term care homes and medical communities use what is called a "Green Form" (note that it is not always on green colored paper) or "Levels of Care" form, which include the following options:

- Full resuscitation: Medical personnel will do everything possible to provide life-sustaining procedures to save the person.

- Health maintenance: No CPR will be administered but the person will be provided with medical help in an intensive care unit (ICU) to sustain the person's health.

- Supportive and comfort care: The person will not receive CPR or be admitted to ICU, but hospitalization and treatment are an option to manage the situation or increase the person's comfort level.

Most doctor clinics have some form of living will, and if they don't, you can ask the doctor where to find more information. In our situation, the Green Form was provided by the doctor and he discussed all the options with my mom and me. When Mom decided on the level of care she wanted, she signed the form. The doctor enacted the form by signing and dating it.

Your parent's living will should be kept somewhere that it can be easily found in an emergency. When researching this section of this book, I contacted old friend Travis Asplund, who is now an EMT-P in Calgary, Alberta. He suggested talking to the EMS in your jurisdiction to find out if it has a program in place for medical emergencies.

"In our area we have a program called the Capsule of Life®. On a specific form, the person records his or her health issues, medication list, and emergency contacts, which provides paramedics with crucial information during an emergency. The form is placed in a plastic capsule and secured underneath the top shelf on the right-hand side of the person's refrigerator. A bright orange decal is placed on the front of the fridge to alert EMS to the capsule," Asplund said.

I contacted the Emergency Medical Services (EMS) Foundation for more information about the Capsule of Life®. The capsule is used when people cannot provide their own medical information, which is ideal for senior citizens, chronically ill persons, and those who live alone and have a medical condition. It's a great program that provides pertinent health and emergency contact information.

It also provides a consistency in that the document provided by the EMS Foundation is the same for every person who uses it, which means, medical personnel can quickly locate the important information on the document during an emergency, and they know where to look for the document (i.e., the refrigerator).

In my personal opinion, I believe the EMS Foundation's Capsule of Life® should be used across North America. If every jurisdiction used the same procedure to find important documents, it could help medical personnel locate information quickly and save many lives.

For more information about the Capsule of Life®, please go to www. emsfoundation.ca.

CHAPTER 6

Finances and Fraud Protection

"In order to plan for financial needs during the course of Alzheimer's disease, you'll need to consider all the costs you might face now and in the future."

— ALZHEIMER'S ASSOCIATION

Before Mom moved home with us, the first sign of her problems with finances came when she called to tell me she couldn't find a huge chunk of her savings. After some investigation I discovered Mom's bank had helped her set up new accounts with better savings and interest rates. The bank had closed the old accounts and transferred the money into the new accounts. Mom was still trying to use her old bank card, check book, and account number.

As was mentioned in previous chapters, you will need to keep detailed records of your parent's finances. If anyone ever questions your work with the finances, the detailed records (in your *Alzheimer's Planner for Caregivers*) will give you proof of what you have been doing and why. Again, I will emphasize that your parent's money is his or hers, *not* yours to do with what you like.

Your first step is to find out which banks your parent deals with and find all the accounts. I organized Mom's accounts into two separate accounts. One was for her savings, big purchases, and automatic bill withdrawals. The other account was for her spending money for when she went out to eat and general shopping. I keep a maximum amount of $1,000 in her spending account so that if someone tries to con Mom or her bank card is stolen, there is not a lot of money in the account that can be stolen from her.

You can set up a maximum withdrawal feature that only allows up to say, $500 per day to be withdrawn. However, if the bank card is stolen and you don't know about it for days or weeks, then whoever stole the card could be withdrawing the daily amount every day until the account is drained dry. Talk to your parent's bank and find out what they suggest in order to protect your parent's money.

Set up automatic withdrawals and deposits so that banking is easier on both you and your parent. Make sure you check the account at least once a month to see what is being automatically withdrawn and if it is the correct amount. Also check if he or she is receiving the proper deposits for pensions and the like.

In the US, the National Council on the Aging (NCOA) provides information on eligibility for discounts on property taxes, health care, and utility bills (benefitscheckup.org). You can also contact the Eldercare Locator (eldercare.gov), provided by the Administration on Aging, which lists social services for the elderly such as home health care.

1. Setting up a Joint Bank Account

I set up both of Mom's bank accounts as joint accounts. This way I don't have to take the Power of Attorney with me every time I have questions for the bank. It also saves me a lot of explaining in regards to why I want information about Mom's accounts.

Every month I can go online and check Mom's accounts to make sure there isn't any abnormal activity. You will need to keep on top of your parent's finances so make sure you are using your *Alzheimer's Planner for Caregivers* to document expenditures. Keep receipts for everything in a file or box so you have the information in case anyone ever questions you about the finances.

If you have siblings or other family members who are concerned about your parent's finances, have a family meeting and explain what you are doing. Your family may not agree with setting up a joint account because other family members may think you will try to use your parent's money for your own spending. I must emphasize again, your parent's money is his or her money, not yours. You should never ever take or "borrow" from your parent's account. Note that your siblings or any other concerned family member can get a court order at any time requiring you to provide the financial records of your parent. When it comes to your parent's finances, you will need to keep accurate records because if there are any discrepancies, you could be in a lot trouble and may even get charged with financial abuse leading to a criminal record.

If anyone in your family is opposed to you having a joint bank account with your parent, or any other joint assets such as a home or vehicle, you should contact a lawyer. The lawyer can create a Statement of Intention, which is a legal document that specifies what to do with assets in joint possession. Normally, a surviving joint account holder will take over the account after the other joint owner dies; however, a Statement of Intention can protect the deceased's wishes of what to do with the joint account or joint asset.

2. Taxes

Keep all medical receipts because anything that isn't covered by medical insurance may be deductible when you file your parent's taxes. This includes medical prescriptions and necessary medical devices such as wheelchairs, walkers, hearing aids, or crutches. The cost of dental treatments such as x-rays, fillings, and dentures may also be tax deductible.

For your own tax purposes as the caregiver, you may be able to deduct renovation costs that are necessary for your parent to reside in your home safely. This may include wheelchair ramps, grab bars for the tub and shower, or railings. If you find you are spending a lot in gas by driving your parent to appointments, this may also be deductible.

You may be able to get a disability tax credit, so talk to your tax authority or accountant to find out if this is possible for your situation.

Depending on your parent's annual income, you may also be able to claim your parent as a dependent. In this situation, the person must be related to you (in-laws are considered related). Again, talk to the IRS, the CRA, or an accountant to find out more about tax breaks. If your parent has a big estate, consider hiring an accountant and/or a financial planner to help you get and stay organized.

3. Debts

If your parent has been having trouble for a while in understanding his or her finances, you may discover debts have piled up. You will need to get these paid or set up payment plans. Go through every single bill your parent has and find out if they have been paid.

If there are large interest charges, talk to the companies to find out if they offer payment plans. Some companies will put a hold on the interest if they know they are now going to be paid what they are owed.

You don't want to get your parent moved and then have nasty bill collectors calling your home and harassing your parent, especially if you are not there to take the call. In Canada, you can contact Consumer Credit Counseling Services (www.creditcounsellingcanada.ca) to help you negotiate with the debt collectors.

Most people don't want to claim bankruptcy; however, if your parent's debt situation is out of control, this may be your only option.

Gather all your parent's credit cards and get them paid off. Once they are paid off, cancel them if they are not necessary. I found there was no need for Mom to have credit cards to rack up debt. Instead she could use her savings for anything she wanted to buy. Credit cards can attract scam artists, so not having any is a good way to protect your parent.

Create a list of outstanding loans, bills, and debts and a schedule of when they are due. Consult this schedule regularly so that you know they are being paid and to check if there are any discrepancies with the payments.

I also highly recommend contacting both TransUnion and Equifax to get a credit check. The reports can provide you with valuable information such as what credit cards are currently active under your parent's name. (For more information read section **5.**)

4. Benefits

Apply for any and all benefits that you can for your parent. Taking care of another person can be extremely expensive depending on the amount of medical care your parent needs. There are many government programs for those who have low income and are in need of supplemental support to survive.

To find out more about government programs for low-income elderly adults, contact your local seniors' organization, the Alzheimer Society or Alzheimer's Association, and local government departments.

5. Fraud Protection

A couple of months after transferring Mom's accounts and setting up automatic withdrawal and deposits, a suspicious phone caller contacted Mom's boyfriend in Saskatchewan. He gave the caller Mom's new phone number and the person began calling for Mom. I took the phone call and I was instantly suspicious when she said she was calling from Canada Pension Plan (CPP). My inner alarm bells were ringing loud and clear as she tried to pressure me by saying "Your Mom won't get her CPP payments if you don't give me her bank account number." I eventually hung up on the caller. I immediately called CPP and followed through with all the steps necessary to protect Mom.

Because of the *Alzheimer's Planner for Caregivers*, I was able to look up all the CPP calls I previously made, which confirmed my suspicions that the mystery caller was a scammer.

If you suspect someone is trying to scam your parent, take the person's phone number and name, then find the real phone number for who the person is claiming to represent and call the real organization. I had the real number for CPP in my Planner and I called them and explained what had happened. No call to us was in CPP's records so they put a note in the account explaining how someone was trying to defraud Mom. The CPP representative also suggested I call the Canadian Anti-Fraud Centre (www.antifraudcentre-centreantifraude.ca) as well as the local police to report it.

In the United States, you can report a suspected fraud to the Federal Trade Commission (FTC), as well as to your state's Attorney General. You should also contact your local police department as well as reporting it to your state's adult protective services agency.

When reporting suspicious calls, you will need to provide the phone number of the caller, the name (if possible), and the time and date the person called.

I went one step further and applied for a credit check with both Trans Union and Equifax as well as putting a fraud alert on Mom's files so that no one could try to open a credit card or get a loan under Mom's name. If you are requesting a fraud alert, you will need to provide the following information to TransUnion and Equifax:

- Cover letter explaining the situation and requesting a fraud alert
- Address (old and new) and phone number
- Date of birth
- Signature

If you know your parent's finances well, what you know will go a long way in protecting your parent.

CHAPTER 7
Understanding the Disease

"The sun shines different ways in summer and winter. We shine different ways in the seasons of our lives."

— TERRI GUILLEMETS

Your parent will be going through a variety of emotions, especially if he or she was recently diagnosed with Alzheimer's disease (AD). Some emotions you and your loved will feel include denial, anger, anxiety, guilt, frustration, sadness, and depression. Being open and talking about the disease can help the person work through his or her emotions as well as help you work through your own emotions. If your loved one is overwhelmed with anxiety and/or depression, talk to his or her doctor because he or she may need medication to help him or her feel calmer.

The Alzheimer Society booklet "Shared Experiences: Suggestions for those with Alzheimer Disease" suggests that talking to others about AD "can help you and others come to terms with the diagnosis. It can open the door for people to offer you social and emotional support."

Your parent's behavior makes sense to your parent; however, it may not always make sense to you, the caregiver. If your parent is acting out, it is for a reason and you will need to figure out what is causing the behavior.

Your loved one's understanding of time may be different now. For example, you may have had a conversation three days earlier and suddenly your parent will pick up where the conversation left off. You may be confused and not understand what your parent is trying to say to you because he or she may have wanted to add something to the previous conversation but forgot, and now is just remembering.

Note that people with Alzheimer's are keenly aware of body language of those around them. For example, if Sheila and I are frustrated even if it has nothing to do with Mom, she knows right away we are frustrated and it can affect her mood for the rest of the day — sometimes even a few days. While we've long forgotten why we were frustrated, or that we were frustrated at all, Mom can get stuck in a groove reliving that moment.

Learn as much as you can about the disease. The more you know, the easier it will be to care for your loved one. Contact the Alzheimer Society or Alzheimer Association for more information.

1. Your Parent Has Rights

Your parent has rights so make sure you respect the following:

- Treat him or her with dignity, compassion, and respect.
- Treat him or her as an adult and as an individual.
- To be informed about his or her diagnosis.
- Given proper medical care.
- Live in a place that is safe and comfortable.
- Encouraged to engage in meaningful activities that suit his or her abilities and interests.
- Be involved in the community (e.g., working, volunteering, and attending functions such as religious services or celebrations).
- Be outdoors and active on a regular basis.
- To be properly cared for and loved.
- Involved in decision making.

When possible, talk to your parent about important decisions. Including him or her in decision making can give the person a form of independence and keep him or her involved. I remind Mom often, "I will be honest with you about everything and explain things to you. I know you may not remember this discussion but I want to get your opinion before I move forward. Just know that I care about what you want and I will do my best to make it happen." It's very important to help fulfill the wishes of your parent.

Don't make promises that you can't keep. Be realistic when talking with your parent. You will constantly need to adapt to new moods and situations as the disease progresses so making promises you can't keep can lead to your parent becoming upset and not trusting you.

You will need to find a balance of what you think is a risk and what is not. You don't want your parent to feel like a prisoner. You will have to learn to see the person as he or she is today, and not as the person you have known him or her to be in the past.

When your parent is in a talkative mood, listen to him or her. If your loved one is discussing memories, ask if you can write down some of the information so that you have those memories for your family in the future. It may also come in handy if you are looking for topics to reminisce about with your parent.

Find out what your parent likes and dislikes. In our family, we know the mere mention of cucumbers sets Mom off into the story of why she refuses to eat cucumbers (she ate too many cucumbers when she was five and it made her sick). If Mom orders a salad in a restaurant, we are sure to tell the server to make sure no cucumbers are included with the salad; otherwise, Mom gets turned off her meal and sometimes seeing cucumbers triggers a bad mood.

2. Person-Centered Care

As you learn more about the disease you may come across the term "person-centered care." This means providing "integrated care, being respectful of and responsive to the person with dementia, family, significant others, and network of support — [his or her] perspectives, needs, values, and choices. This approach involves the person with dementia and family as partners in decision-making processes, and ensures integration of the person with dementia and families into the care team in order to maintain optimal, evolving care." From the Alzheimer Society of Canada — Older Adult Abuse and Dementia: A Literature Review; prepared by MaryLou Harrigan, EdD Research Consultant.

The concept of person-centered care is meant to help the person participate fully in his or her environment and to provide him or her with the following:

- Dignity
- Respect
- Information sharing
- Participation
- Collaboration

It's important to remember that your parent is a person with a disease. Listen to what your parent is telling you, even if it is repeated several times. The person wants to be heard and not ignored. Whatever he or she is saying is important to him or her, so listen.

In our situation I always tell Mom, we have an open-honesty policy. Even though she can't always remember what is discussed, I get her opinion so that I know how to go about whatever it is I'm doing for her. We don't tip-toe around the disease; we discuss it and work through the difficult moments together. In essence, we work with the limitations of the disease and not against it.

By asking Mom's opinion, she feels she is participating in her care and decision making. By working together, we help Mom to feel she is a valued member of our family as well as it gives us a chance to understand what she is going through, which helps us to provide better care for her.

3. Health problems

Be aware of any ailments your loved one tries to describe. He or she may not know how to describe the problem, but it could be something serious.

Be alert for pain cues. For example, Mom had to have IV meds administered by a nurse and the nurse pushed the syringe too quickly, which caused Mom a great deal of pain. She couldn't voice her pain, but her facial features scrunched up into a look of agony. The next time a nurse administered IV meds, I told the nurse to do it slow because it hurts Mom if done too quickly.

Never undermine your parent by telling him or her that the problem isn't serious. If he or she is trying to describe something to you, take notes and when you see the doctor next, bring up your parent's concerns.

4. Communication

As the disease progresses, you may find your parent has trouble communicating. Try not to finish your parent's sentences, unless he or she says that's okay, because this may upset him or her. You are taking away a piece of your parent's independence when you begin speaking for him or her.

As the disease evolves, you will need to adapt to the changes your parent is experiencing. In the book, *Coach Broyles' Playbook for Alzheimer's Caregivers: A Practical Tips Guide*, by Frank Broyles, the author says, "It is now your job to change how you talk with her to match what she can understand."

There was a situation where Mom kept asking me to buy Liquid Paper for her. So I got her a bottle. Two days later she asked me again for the correction fluid. I figured she must have misplaced the bottle I had brought to her. So, I bought her another bottle. A few more days go by and she wants another one! This time, I took her to her room and showed her the two bottles sitting on her desk. She looked at me confused and then pointed to her face. After some discussion, we finally got to what she really wanted — concealer, which is a cosmetic that covers up blemishes.

Always pay attention to your parent's body language. I know when Mom is feeling uncomfortable because she begins to curl into herself. What I mean by that is she balls her hands into tight fists and holds them close to her body. If she is sitting, she will also pull her legs up and in front of her.

Don't cut your parent off, even if this is the 10th, 20th, or 30th time of the day you have heard the same comment. Sometimes, all it takes is to change the topic or give him or her an activity to do.

If your parent is asking to go "home," it may not even be his or her former home that he or she wants to be. It could be a childhood home that has long since been demolished. One lecture I attended, the speaker said, "Sometimes home to a person with Alzheimer's may not even exist on our physical plane." Home may just be somewhere the person remembers as feeling comfortable and safe but physically there is nowhere you can take your parent that has that feeling of "home."

5. Simplify

It can be hard for a person with AD to understand what you are saying, especially if you are talking fast or giving too many instructions at once. If you ask your parent a question, give him or her time to answer. You may need to repeat the question if your parent forgets what he or she was trying to say.

Keep your instructions simple by using small words and avoiding slang. Begin with one step then move on to the next when your parent has completed the first step.

If your parent likes to do dishes but has trouble figuring out where to put the dishes when they are dry, put sticky notes on the cupboards directing where to put glasses, plates, and bowls. Ask your parent if he or she is okay with you doing this so as not to offend him or her. It may be a big relief for him or her to see the cupboards labeled.

At the end of each day, mark off the date on the calendar so when your parent gets up in the morning, he or she knows the date.

Hang recent pictures of family and friends. You can even label the pictures with names or have a short write up about the event where the picture was taken. This can help your parent remember who is currently involved in his or her life.

6. Dealing with Problem Behaviors

People with Alzheimer's don't always follow the same logic as the caregiver. This is why it is important to try to understand what your parent may be trying to tell you. As the disease progresses, your loved one may not know how to translate if he or she is in pain or upset. You can buy "Emotion Cards," which display different moods such as happy or sad or angry and they can help your parent "show" what mood he or she is feeling.

Some people with AD become suspicious and paranoid as the disease progresses. Your parent may misplace an item and then begin yelling at you for stealing the prized possession. Don't take the negative comments towards you personally; instead see if you can help the person find the misplaced item. You can also try to distract the person with something else until you find the missing item.

Changes in routine can cause considerable upset for the person with AD so try to stick to routines and schedules as much as possible.

Do not ever argue or yell at the person when he or she is in a bad mood. Instead, try to lighten the mood or change the topic, if possible. You may find it difficult when your parent is going through a bad spell; however, consider how hard this disease is on him or her. It's frustrating for the person because he or she can no longer express himself or herself like he or she used to do.

Try positive reinforcement such as a smile or a gentle hug when your parent is feeling down. However, if you believe your parent may strike out and hit you, back away and give him or her time to cool down. It may be as simple as putting on soothing music or gently talking to the person. If you stay calm during a really bad episode, this can help defuse the situation.

After a bad episode, you may be able to talk with your parent and discover what triggered the mood swing. Try not to push your parent into the conversation; if he or she doesn't want to talk about it, you will need to let the topic go, or you may even try the conversation again at another time.

One of the tricks Sheila uses to get Mom out of a foul mood is to buy her flowers. Mom loves to compliment the flowers and she takes care of them by adding water and removing the dead leaves and petals. Flowers are a great distraction her from a bad mood.

6.1 Shadowing

You may find your parent follows you from room to room. This behavior is called shadowing. It may give your parent comfort to be around you constantly but for you, you may find it slightly distracting!

If you notice your parent is shadowing you, sometimes you just need to sit still for a short time and visit with your parent to ease his or her fears of abandonment. Other times you may be able to direct your parent to an activity; maybe the reason for the shadowing is that the person is bored but doesn't know what to do. You may also be able to distract the person by getting another family member to visit with your parent while you get what you need to get done around your home.

6.2 Sundowning

Sundowning is a term that refers to people with Alzheimer's who go into a state of confusion and agitation at the end of the day and into the night. It may be caused by a disruption to the body's internal clock due to the disease.

Fatigue, low lighting, and increased shadows can increase the likelihood of sundowning. If your parent is sleeping a lot during the day, but he or she is up and restless at night, you may need to get the person into more daytime activities so he or she is more likely to sleep at night. Also, reduce or stop caffeine intake and sugar during the afternoon and evening. Having a consistent schedule of when the person goes to bed and wakes up in the morning can help as well.

6.3 Inappropriate language and topics

Sheila and I were at a loss at what to do with Mom when she said inappropriate things in front of the grandkids such as swearing in front of my preteen nephew. There was one uncomfortable instance where what Mom said was completely inappropriate in front of my teenage niece and her boyfriend — so shocking that it stopped the conversation. Because of the silence that followed her comment, Mom just about burst into tears from the embarrassment. I tried to smooth over the situation by making a funny comment, which helped everyone give a chuckle and removed Mom from the spotlight.

Sheila and I realized we had to talk to the kids about Grandma and why she sometimes may say things that aren't exactly appropriate for them to hear. This is where books about Alzheimer's geared for children can come in handy.

Try to smooth the situation with humor because scolding your parent is not acceptable. He or she won't always know what was said or how it came across to those who heard it.

6.4 Problems with eating

In my research, and by observing Mom, I came across many problems with a person with AD either overeating or refusing to eat. In Mom's situation, she would refuse to eat because she didn't feel hungry. How I convinced her to eat is by explaining to her that her pills needed to be taken with food. Once she began eating, she was fine and would continue to eat. The disease has robbed her of the ability to feel hunger, but that doesn't mean that her body is not hungry.

Another problem we had is if we let Mom dish up her own plate, she would take a miniscule amount and she could not be convinced to eat a reasonable amount of food. To combat this, I began plating her meals. Again, once she began eating, she would eat everything on the plate.

One expert suggested that people with AD are more likely to eat from plates that have color (i.e., not white plates). Both Sheila and I have colored plates that we use, but it hasn't seemed to stimulate Mom's appetite. However, that doesn't mean it won't work for others.

I came across stories where a person with AD will eat a whole bowl of potatoes or other food if it is put in front of him or her. If your parent is overeating, try dishing up his or her plate with a reasonable amount of food and do not leave out excess food.

Mom came from a time that no food was wasted so Sheila found out rather quickly that Mom got upset if she saw Sheila cleaning out expired food from the fridge. I even caught Mom digging out the food from the garbage because she felt it was such a waste. Now, when Sheila cleans out the fridge, she does it when Mom is out of the house. She empties the fridge and right away throws out the garbage so Mom doesn't see the rotten expired food in the garbage.

Even though Mom claims she is never hungry, I found a rotting banana in her underwear drawer. My teenage niece, Ashleigh, is usually the last one up at night and she began to notice Mom sneaking into the kitchen and grabbing muffins or fruit to take to bed with her. Sheila and I now encourage her to eat snacks during the day and evening because we assume she must be feeling hunger during the night. Since Mom loves sweets and fruit, by offering her a granola bar or peach before bed she willingly accepts it and it seems to help prevent her from stashing food in her room. The problem with stashing food is that it can be forgotten, which leads to a rotten mess to clean up later!

It's not that we don't feed Mom enough at mealtimes, or that she can't go in the kitchen any time to grab food, instead I believe stashing food is something she did when she was a kid growing up in a very poor home. I also believe that is why she becomes upset when Sheila cleans out the fridge.

6.5 Problems with clothing

Your parent may want to wear the same clothing day in and day out. This can be a problem because clothes do get dirty, and underwear should be changed daily. You may have to buy a few of the same outfits so that when your parent takes off the clothing, they go in a laundry basket right away and the "same" outfit is still in the closet for the next day.

Monday morning we have a routine where Mom gets up and has a bath. If I don't catch her before she's dressed, she flat-out refuses to take a bath. While she is in the bathtub, I go through her closet and find the clothes she wore the previous week. (She always rehangs the clothing she has worn.) I get everything into the laundry machine before she gets out of the tub. This way she doesn't return to her room and put on dirty clothing.

As Mom's disease progressed, she began having trouble sequencing her clothing properly. She would put her bra over her shirt and then add a sweater on top of the shirt and bra. How I discovered she was having this problem is that she kept fidgeting with her sweater. She admitted her bra wasn't fitting right and that's when she realized she had her bra over her shirt and that it wasn't the right way to wear it. After that, if I noticed her fidgeting in a similar way, I would ask if she had her bra on correctly and she would check.

Another problem with clothing is the person may not know how to dress for the weather. In winter, your parent may try wearing a t-shirt and shoes without ice gripping on the soles. Or in summer, he or she insists on wearing layers of sweaters. A little trick is to change around the clothing in the closet during the season changes. For example, moving the sweaters to the back of the closet in spring and moving forward long-sleeved lighter shirts to the front, eventually as summer moves in, put the t-shirts at the front.

For example, when Mom moved home with us, I gave her a fall jacket that was long and black. As winter set it, I gave her a similar but thicker long black jacket and put the other fall jacket in the back of her closet. She didn't notice the transition so it went smoothly.

Shoes were another problem because Mom used to wear high heels all the time but as she got older, her balance wasn't as good as it once was. I substituted her high heels with similar colored flats with good grips and made sure they were still fancy. She enjoyed having the new shoes and because they were still fancy, she could feel elegant while I felt comfort knowing she was safe.

6.6 Problems with bathing

When I was growing up, Mom seemed to always be in the bathtub. She loved her baths! It was a way for her to calm down at the end of a stressful day. Nowadays, Mom loathes bathing. Even though there are three bathrooms at Sheila's, Mom doesn't want to tie up the bathroom! That's why on Monday morning, when no one but Mom and I are at home, I can convince her to take a bath.

Some days I really struggle with Mom because she outright refuses to take a bath and will even go so far as to tell me, "I just had a bath yesterday." This is one of the many reasons a Memory Book is so important. I always ask her to write in her book when she has had a bath so that when she is adamant she has taken a bath, I tell her she should read back in her Memory Book. When she discovers she hasn't bathed the previous day, she's mad but she will take a bath. If I couldn't prove to her that she hasn't bathed, it would be an all-out war of refusal.

For whatever reason, bathing is one of the hardest things for caregivers to deal with when it comes to a person with AD. I suggest scheduling a specific day of the week as bath day. The time of day will depend on what suits your parent, not you. Early in the morning works best for Mom, but for your parent, it may be just before bed or midafternoon.

You will need to set aside a couple of hours for the whole process such as getting the bath ready and waiting for your parent to prepare for the bath. I find Mom procrastinates so as I'm pouring the water she'll eat breakfast, do the dishes, pick out her outfit for the day, and brush her teeth.

A side note about bathing. People with Alzheimer's don't always feel temperature properly. I always check the dish water and tub water before Mom dips into them. You can buy anti-scalding devices for your taps, which I strongly recommend.

One of the ways I convince Mom to take a bath is by reminding her that we are going somewhere that day or the next so I know she will want to look her best. To make it easier on her, I lay out a fresh towel and facecloth as well as soap, shampoo, and conditioner.

You could also use a reward system such as taking your parent for ice cream or for a drive after the bath is done. It creates something to look forward to after doing something he or she doesn't want to do.

Adding special touches to the bath can also help. For Mom, she loves bath bubbles so I make sure to add a lot. I've heard others say they add toys such as a rubber ducky or sailboat. Toys can make the person feel comfortable and may even remind him or her about a good bath experience as a child.

If your parent just won't bath, ask a doctor for recommendations of what to do. If your parent listens to the doctor, you may be able to get the doctor to write on a prescription pad "Bathe Mondays and Thursdays every week." Having that as a reminder from a professional may encourage your parent to take a bath.

CHAPTER 8

Activities

"Keeping occupied and stimulated can improve quality of life for the person with dementia as well as those around them."

ALZHEIMER SOCIETY (UK WEBSITE)

You will need to find meaningful activities for your loved one to help keep him or her feel involved, and it will help to keep him or her socially and physically active. You may find your loved one becomes restless so taking a drive or going window shopping will help reduce the person's boredom. Just going to the movies makes Mom feel like it was a fantastic day even if that is all we did.

The activities should be age appropriate and meaningful to your parent. To find appropriate activities for your parent, focus on his or her remaining skills. Doing activities that he or she is having trouble with can cause frustration and trigger bad mood swings. Pay attention to your parent's nonverbal cues so you know whether or not he or she is enjoying the activity.

Social activities give the person a connection to others so if you have a seniors' center that provides some of the activities listed in this chapter, encourage your parent to join. Physical activities help keep a person active and healthy. Cognitive activities such as card and memory games can help exercise the brain and provide the person with mental stimulation. Work together with your parent to build a list of things he or she wants to do that includes a variety of social, physical, and cognitive activities.

Find out what activities are important to your parent. Will there be challenges for your parent? If so, can you adjust the activity so that it is not overwhelming or dangerous for your parent (e.g., give the person a smaller area to attend to in the garden).

Mom was never one to have hobbies so at first Sheila and I were at a loss of what to do with her. She loved reading, but that was a solo activity. We wanted to do more social activities with her which would engage her in conversation and give her a reason to go outside the house. This chapter describes some of the activities we found worked for Mom as well some activities suggested by the Alzheimer Society.

1. Alzheimer Café

If you're in a location where an Alzheimer Café is hosted each month, take your parent to the meetings. Conny Schipper, former Manager of Client Services and Programs, Alzheimer Society of Alberta and Northwest Territories, explains, "The Alzheimer Café is a great place for families living with Alzheimer's disease or related dementia to socialize, share ideas, and gain information in an informal and safe setting."

The first Alzheimer Café began in the Netherlands in 1997 and it is just now catching on in North America. The café provides a wonderful environment for those with Alzheimer's and their caregivers to go to discuss the disease and also to enjoy the company of others in similar situations.

At our café, Schipper did a fantastic job of booking guest speakers such as nurses and other professionals who discuss the disease. The guests are not always medical professionals, but musicians and poets. The meetings are interactive so everyone is encouraged to participate in the activities and discussions by asking questions and sharing stories.

The event is hosted by the Round Street Café, which donates tasty treats and good coffee for the event. Our family enjoys going to the café and meeting other caretakers and those with AD because it gives us a feeling that we are not alone on this journey. The environment is comfortable and jovial so it makes it a monthly treat for Mom. It is a wonderful place to socialize.

If there isn't an Alzheimer's Café in your area, talk to your local Alzheimer Society. You may find that they are more than willing, with a little help, to get one started in your area.

2. Pet Love

Many people love animals but for whatever reason cannot have a pet in their home. Going to a pet store that lets customers interact with the animals can be a fun adventure for your loved one. If the employees aren't busy, they are more than happy to pull a bunny out of its cage so your parent can pet the animal. The pet store by my place has chinchillas, guinea pigs, and bunnies which can be petted and held. The best thing about this activity is it doesn't cost anything to browse in a pet store.

Take your time when you go through the store with your parent. The experience may trigger happy memories of pets from his or her past. Enjoy the stories your parent tells and enjoy the time you are spending with your parent.

Mom enjoyed whistling at the parrot and other various birds. And the birds enjoyed the interaction as well!

You can also take your parent to the zoo or a petting zoo if there is one nearby. Maybe you have a friend or family member that lives on a farm so a day trip to visit the farm animals will be a good experience for your parent.

If a dog show is coming to your city, ask your parent if he or she would like to attend the event. Seeing these beautiful animals on display can be a delight for your loved one.

Find animal movies or YouTube videos and share the experience with your parent. Mom and I spent an afternoon on a snowy day watching YouTube videos of pets doing funny and cute things. It was a good afternoon filled with lots of laughter.

Animals can trigger memories and if a person is having a bad day, pet therapy may be able to bring some sunshine to an otherwise gray day for your loved one. Lynn Crackel volunteers with her dog, Logan, who is part of the St. John Ambulance Therapy Dog Program. She has seen firsthand how pets can help those with physical and mental disabilities:

"As soon as Logan enters the home he is immediately recognized and acknowledged (many patients don't recognize me or know my name). The residents' smiles light up and their hands are extended as soon as Logan enters a room or walks down a hallway. Some of the seniors don't recognize him from week to week, but they still love to see him and I usually get to hear a short story about their childhood with their pets. Seeing Logan always invokes memories for the patients from their past and the seniors love to talk about the pets they had when they were younger; the pets are always remembered with great fondness.

"When meeting seniors who don't have a lot of mobility, or who may suffer from dementia, I can see the extra effort that they put in just to have a bit of time petting Logan. They love the feeling of a floppy ear and a furry chest. It's the pure joy they get out of touching a creature that returns their love and attention."

Heather Mueller, BSW, RSW, AAT, and author of *Start & Run a Pet Business*, provides pet therapy to seniors' groups and she had this to say:

"When working with seniors who have been diagnosed with either Alzheimer's or dementia, Animal Assisted Activities or Therapies can be very beneficial. Research shows interaction with animals can have a positive effect on dopamine and serotonin levels as well as blood pressure and heart rate.

"Many seniors' recreation services in Canada have incorporated some form of Animal Assisted Activities into their programing. Being a mental health animal assisted therapist since 2004, I have witnessed many positive reactions to animal interactions when working with seniors over the years. One of the most fascinating reactions I have witnessed is the ability for some seniors suffering through various effects of short-term memory loss, to remember not only the animals I bring to visit, but their names as well. Even under the ravages of Alzheimer's or dementia many of my clients have astounded residential staff by completely changing in function and personality the minute an animal is presented. Though there is no concrete scientific explanation as to why this occurs, it is my observation that despite other details being eroded from their memories, their love of animals enables them to hold onto that connection."

3. Shopping

If your parent doesn't mind crowds, you may want to go window shopping or just shopping in general. Going to an interesting store that sells items on the unusual side may be an interesting experience. We have a couple of stores in our area that sell unique inexpensive jewelry and vintage fashion accessories. Mom loves looking through the bobbles and trinkets on display. The store turns over its products monthly so every time we go in the store there is something new and interesting to look at.

Taking your parent to antique stores or second-hand stores can trigger memories of items he or she grew up with. It's similar to going to a museum in that he or she can relive his or her memories with you.

Asking your parent to shop with you for gifts and cards for special occasions is also a nice way to include your parent in decision making. If your parent doesn't like crowds, or he or she finds them overwhelming, go shopping early in the morning when it is less busy. During Christmas time, try to shop for presents at the beginning of December so your parent doesn't have to fight his or her way through crowds and long lineups.

Maybe your parent likes to make crafts. If so, a weekly or monthly trip to the craft store to replenish supplies may be a fun outing that your parent can plan for by preparing a list of the things he or she needs to complete his or her projects. Summer craft fairs may be an ideal place to take your parent. Even Flea Markets may provide interesting items for your parent to use for hobby projects.

If your parent likes to cook, take your parent to a Farmers' Market. Walking around in the open air and talking with the merchants is a great way for your parent to socialize. The bonus is he or she may find interesting foods to add to his or her recipes, which will make dinners at your place a surprise and a treat!

4. Family Celebrations and Dining Out

If your parent is always cooking, give him or her a break and go out to eat. In our situation, I don't cook so we get tired of having sandwiches and soup for lunch. I found a unique place called The Jasmine Room, which is a boutique and tea room. When entering the business we pause to look at all the antiques and new unique items the store has for sale. Then we settle in to a homemade meal. Mom loves going to this restaurant because it is small and never overly crowded. She can look at the antique items displayed on the walls as she eats and once in a while she will discover an old tea cup or hat on a shelf that reminds her of her childhood.

Your parent may like a certain type of food such as Italian or Chinese. You could order in and have a movie night. Make it a theme night by renting *The Godfather* while serving pasta from your favorite local Italian restaurant!

In this day and age of blended families, you may have a lot of step-family who your parent doesn't know. If there is a big family event such as a milestone birthday, graduation, or wedding, don't exclude your parent with AD. Your parent is part of your family so, if possible, encourage him or her to participate in the preparation for the event.

When my parents divorced more than 25 years ago, they parted ways on bad terms. As the years went by, family functions were always awkward because we never knew how to deal with our parents being in the same room. Now, as the Alzheimer's has progressed, Mom has left behind any animosity she held towards Dad so family functions are less awkward.

If your parents are divorced, and there is a big family function on the horizon, talk with both of your parents and find out how to make the situation comfortable for both of them. It may be that they need to sit on opposite sides of the room. If you're lucky like we are, maybe enough time has passed so bad feelings have been forgotten and everyone has moved on.

5. Walking and Driving Tours

If your parent is fit, and he or she enjoys walking, go on a walking tour. Some areas have grave tours that describe well-known past citizens that influenced the city or town to become what it is today.

You could also take a guided tour of a mine, bird sanctuary, or botanical garden. During Christmas, there may be an opportunity to do a Christmas lights tour. Seeing the bright lights can bring back memories of childhood holidays.

Look around to see what tours are offered in your area. Even just a simple car ride around a historic neighborhood can be a fun outing. Sometimes we ignore the beauty in our own backyards and spend money to travel far away. However, you may not have the luxury of traveling far away, so be a tourist in your own area. You may be surprised at the interesting things you find.

If you live by the ocean, or any body of water, there are usually parks close by that have nice smooth walkways. You want to make sure that your parent will not be exhausted or hurt during the excursion so only choose activities that your parent is physically comfortable doing. The terrain should be simple making sure it is not too strenuous or that it doesn't have obstacles that can cause trips or falls.

When going on long walks, make sure you pack a bag of supplies, even if the walk is only an hour or less. Bring plenty of water, snacks, and bug spray. Make sure your parent has proper walking shoes and if he or she needs a cane or walking stick, bring that as well.

Layers of clothing are also important so your parent doesn't get cold, but he or she can remove the layers if it is too hot. On hot days bring a hat for your parent, and on overcast days bring an umbrella just in case.

Take breaks and sit down on a bench so your parent can rest. During these rest times you may be able to catch sight of a bird or two that intrigues your parent. Walking through a park is a perfect place to watch wildlife and do some bird watching. You may even want to pick up a nature book that includes animals and birds that reside in your area. Make a game of it and see how many creatures in the wild you can find and circle them in the book.

You could also help your parent begin a collection of leaves and flowers during walks in parks or seashells when walking by the ocean. Your parent can glue leaves or flowers into his or her Memory Book.

Mom loves motorcycle rides, so when my brother, Shawn, offered to take her on a ride during a camping trip, she leapt at the opportunity.

Sheila took a picture to remember the moment and sent it to me. Mom was grinning from ear to ear!

If you notice your parent is tired or becoming agitated, take a break. If that doesn't help his or her mood, you may want to cut short the walk and find another activity. Or maybe your parent just wants to go home and nap. Always watch for nonverbal cues to see if your parent is enjoying the outing or not.

6. Music

Research has shown that music is good for people who suffer from AD. We always have the country music station playing softly in the background. I'm not a fan of country music, but I can tolerate it because Mom loves it. When she is reading she finds the music soothing.

One person told me about a situation where a patient in a long-term care facility no longer talked but if a favorite song was played, the patient would sing all the words!

Your parent may enjoy going to concerts and music recitals. If crowds aren't a problem, why not take your parent for a special evening of live music. Some cities, such as Winnipeg, have outdoor music festivals throughout the summer. Some music events are free while others sell inexpensive tickets.

If your parent likes to sing or play an instrument, see if there is a seniors' organization that accepts people into their musical groups. Your parent may be interested in singing in a church choir, so consider talking to your minister about whether or not your parent can join the choir.

It may sound corny, but a family sing-a-long with young grandchildren can brighten your parent's day! If you have a karaoke machine, dust it off and bring it for a night of family fun!

7. Gardening

Gardening can be an activity your parent enjoys. However, make sure the job you assign to your parent is small and easy. You don't want your parent to overexert himself or herself. I find Mom tends to become obsessive-compulsive with a task and won't stop until it is finished, which is neither healthy nor enjoyable for her.

Also, be prepared for the odd mistake when gardening with your parent. For example, Mom said she would hoe my vegetable garden, which never really grows anything but one uncommon herb, sorrel. Unfortunately, Mom hoed my poor sorrel plant beyond repair. I was a little disappointed because it was the only plant I've managed to grow and keep growing year after year, but I expected this might happen. I never said anything to her about it. Instead, I complimented her on doing a wonderful job with the garden.

Going to a greenhouse can be a fun adventure for you and your parent. Give him or her some independence by letting him or her choose some veggies and flowers to take home and plant. It may not be what you want in your garden scheme, but you can redesign your garden the way you like someday when your parent is no longer around. And who knows, maybe your parent's choices will "grow" on you!

More strenuous and potentially dangerous activities such as cutting branches and mowing the lawn should be left to you or your spouse or children. You don't want the activity to hurt your parent and exhaust him or her. Note that activities with your parent are meant to be fun and relaxing and not real "work."

8. Wrapping Presents and Decorating the Home for the Holidays

Holidays can be a fun time of year but families can have routines of how and when they decorate. How you decorate your home and how your parent likes to decorate can be two completely different styles.

For example, I don't decorate at all during the Christmas season. I find it a waste of time because I eventually have to take down the decorations; whereas, Sheila goes all out with a nicely decorated tree and trimmings around the house. Sheila put a lovely fake Christmas bouquet in Mom's room, and a week later Mom was trying to give it to me to take home for a decoration in my house. Since I didn't want to take it home, Mom was going to give it to her best friend. I thought it was something Mom brought with her from Saskatoon, but it was something Sheila had received from a special relative of hers years earlier. When Sheila discovered this, we decided to remove it from Mom's room because for whatever reason, she just didn't want it in there and sooner or later she would have given it to someone if we didn't remove it!

I have a friend who only allows blue, silver, and white decorations in her house during the holidays. That includes the wrapping paper on the presents. I find more and more, people want the perfect catalog designed Christmas decorations. This may not be your parent's style, so let him or her incorporate his or her style into yours so that the festivities are enjoyable for everyone. What is the worst that can happen if a pink-wrapped present ends up under a tree filled with blue, white, and silver decorations?

Mom is a master gift wrapper, so much so, that we all got her to wrap our presents during the holidays. She adds beautiful bows and unique decorations to the gifts, which makes a person not want to open them because they are so beautiful. She would take her time with each gift, but the downside to that is by the time she got it wrapped, she forgot what was in the gift and who it was to and from!

We designed a system where I added sticky notes to the unwrapped gifts saying who the gift was going to and who it was from. She would put the sticky note to the side when she was ready to wrap the present and she would create a name card to put on the gift when it was wrapped. Mom and I laughed and said how funny it would be if Sheila received a gift of boxer shorts while Shawn got some nice perfume!

Wrapping gifts and participating in the decorating of your home can be fun for everyone, especially your parent. Cherish these times together and take lots of pictures to remember the happy festivities.

9. Sports and Exercise

Depending on your parent's motor skills, he or she may still enjoy doing some types of sports such as fishing, golfing, or swimming. If your parent likes family activities such as bowling, why not rent a lane for the evening and have a family night out? Again, watch for nonverbal cues to see if your parent is enjoying the activity, if not, ask if he or she would like to leave and go do something else.

I took Mom to a seniors' aquasize (water aerobics) class; unfortunately, Mom no longer had the coordination to do the simple exercises and stretches so it was frustrating for her and she became increasingly agitated with it. However, taking her just to swim or sit in the hot tub was okay.

You may need to consult with your parent's doctor about what physical activities your parent is capable of doing. Your parent may think he or she is in perfect physical shape, and that may be so, however, his or her coordination may not be what it once was.

Other forms of exercise may include:

- Yoga
- Tai Chi
- Soccer
- Basketball
- Going to the batting cages

- Tennis
- Kayaking or canoeing
- Dancing
- Beanbag toss
- Darts
- Shuffleboard
- Bocce ball
- Lawn bowling
- Croquet

10. Other Activities

There are many activities you can do with your parent. Assess his or her skill level and find out what he or she is interested in doing then do it! If your parent is not having fun, or if he or she is becoming frustrated, put away the activity for a while.

When planning activities, begin with small projects and avoid activities with too many steps. Consider the person's abilities and safety level (e.g., working with woodworking equipment may be too dangerous for your parent).

Here are some other activities your parent may enjoy:

- Quilting, knitting, cross-stitching, or joining a sewing circle
- Attending church services
- Light duties such as cleaning and small fix-up projects
- Woodworking
- Card games (e.g., memory-matching or Go Fish) or board games
- Photography
- Attending a ballet
- Scrapbooking
- Painting (e.g., paint-by-numbers) or drawing
- Joining a book group for seniors
- Playing Bingo

- Going to a movie
- Watching old favorite shows on DVD or Blu-ray
- Watching old family movies or slide shows
- Camping
- Reciting poetry or attending poetry readings
- Writing short stories or memoir-style stories
- Visiting friends and family
- Going to the library
- Creating a scavenger hunt for your family
- Jewelry making
- Pottery making or ceramics
- Going to museums
- Going to art galleries
- Volunteering in the community
- Star or cloud gazing
- Origami
- Reading print and picture books
- Coloring books or velvet coloring posters
- Solving puzzles or word games (e.g., jigsaw or word searches)
- Having a manicure and pedicure (which is also good foot care)

Leave out some activities for your parent so that if he or she is feeling bored, her or she may be more inclined to work on a project. For example, one person I talked to suggested leaving a puzzle partially finished on a table. Every now and again, your parent may see a piece that fits and add it to the puzzle. When the puzzle is complete, remove a few of the pieces and your loved one can accomplish the task of finishing it again.

11. Day Programs for People with Alzheimer's

As the disease progresses you may need to put your parent into programs that have suitable activities for his or her stage of AD. Or maybe you need a couple of days a week away from your parent to catch up on your own life or to prevent caregiver burnout. (See Chapter 10 for more information about self-care for caregivers.) Talk to your local branch of the Alzheimer Society for information about the programs in your area.

After nine months of being with Mom, Monday through Friday from nine until four, working my evening job, and trying to keep up with my freelance deadlines, I was beginning to feel overwhelmed. I was also feeling guilty because Mom would read and nap all day every day when I was unable to spend one-on-one time with her doing activities because I was too busy trying to make my next deadline. I couldn't stop working because I needed a steady income, yet I didn't want to neglect Mom either.

I explained to Mom that I needed to get her in a program for a couple days during the week so she could socialize with others. It wasn't that I was trying to get rid of her, but instead it was for her own well-being. It also would give her some independence away from the family so she could have her very own activity to attend instead of doing only family activities. Explaining it this way to her made her want to go out and meet others as opposed to feeling like she was being shuffled off for the day. She didn't feel like a burden because I explained I wasn't doing this for me but for her. In truth, it was best for both of us, but explaining that it was more for her to meet others made it easier for her to accept it willingly.

In our area, in order to get Mom into a program we had to register for Home Care, which provides services to complement the care provided by family. Home Care is an excellent system that helps families navigate through the complicated medical system. Home Care's mission statement is "to assist individuals of the region to achieve and maintain an optimal level of health, and personal independence." Home Care provides support so people can remain as independent as possible in their own homes and communities as opposed to going into long-term care.

Once we were signed up, a Home-Care nurse (also known as a Case Manager) came by Sheila's home and talked with Mom and I to find out what stage of Alzheimer's she was at. The nurse also coordinated with Mom's doctors so he had an accurate picture of Mom's needs. His job was to assess her situation and then help us find her meaningful activities appropriate to her skill level outside the home environment. A Home-Care nurse can provide valuable information about programs offered for seniors, as well as respite care for caregivers.

In Canada, we have the nonprofit group, Victorian Order of Nurses (VON). This organization provides an adult day center where Mom can go twice a week to socialize with other people with Alzheimer's. Throughout the day she participates in light physical exercises, crafts, and memory games. They provide a home-cooked lunch and a coffee chat time in the afternoon. If Mom is tired, she can curl up in a comfy chair and sleep or read. This is something that breaks up the week for Mom and it gives me time to focus on my work. Every week she looks forward to seeing her new friends and the people who run the program.

The employees at VON are wonderful and they like to keep us, the family, in the loop with any concerns or any good things that happen throughout the day with Mom. I also don't have to worry about her wandering because they keep the facility doors locked so no one ever goes outside without a guardian.

I'm finding it easier to keep on top of my deadlines and my own stress levels have been reduced. When I pick her up from VON at the end of the day, she is all smiles and giggles and excitedly tells me about her day. If she hasn't written anything in her Memory Book, we spend time going over her day and she writes down what she did at VON.

VON also works with Access-a-Ride, which can pick up the person in the morning and drop him or her off in the afternoon. However, not everyone likes to go on the bus. Mom tried the bus a few times but she found it too stressful waiting for the bus because she always assumed she had missed it and then she would panic.

The daily fees for the program are reasonable; however, space is limited so if you feel this is the right program for your parent, you should talk to a VON representative in your area.

You may also want to check out the local seniors' center for programs offered in your area. They may have a similar program to VON that your parent can attend. There may also be day programs in a rehabilitation center for seniors suffering from physical disabilities.

Talk to the Geriatric Specialist, a home-care nurse, or a seniors' center for more information about day programs for seniors with Alzheimer's.

On a side note, never call it "adult daycare" because it is insulting. Your parent is not a child, and should not be treated as such. It's a "day program" or "day center" for seniors or people with Alzheimer's.

CHAPTER 9
Elder Abuse

Elder Abuse: "A single, or repeated act, or lack of appropriate action, occurring within any relationship where there is an expectation of trust which causes harm or distress to an older person."

— WORLD HEALTH ORGANIZATION (WHO)

Older people are vulnerable to abuse, especially those who have cognitive impairments. Elder abuse can be physical, mental, verbal, or financial. People who abuse can be close family members, friends, or even strangers. Some people may not even realize that their actions are abusive.

Intimidation, domination, isolation, and control are all considered elder abuse. Whether it is a single incident or a pattern, abuse is unacceptable. A person with Alzheimer's is entitled to respect, a safe environment, and security.

1. Types of Elder Abuse

Depending on what stage of Alzheimer's and how long the person has been with the abuser, the person may no longer be able to comprehend that he or she is being abused. The abuse may have been in place long before the AD diagnosis or it may have started when the person began showing signs of the disease.

Some victims are aware of the abuse but they are embarrassed or scared to ask for help while others are afraid of being placed in a long-term care facility.

1.1 Emotional and psychological abuse

Emotional abuse can be both verbal and nonverbal. Emotional abusers attack the person's sense of dignity and self-worth by demoralizing, dehumanizing, and intimidating. Types of emotional abuse include:

- Shouting
- Bullying
- Insults
- Criticizing
- Blaming
- Intimidation
- Humiliation
- Threats of violence
- Isolation or ignoring
- Aggressive or taunting behavior
- Using guilt to make the person do something

The victim may show signs of emotional abuse such as the following:

- Feelings of guilt, hopelessness, shame, and/or inadequacy
- Withdrawal from family, friends, and routine activities outside of the home
- Heightened anxiety or discomfort around the suspected abuser
- Increased levels of agitation

1.2 Physical and sexual abuse

Physical abuse means inflicting physical pain, impairment, and/or injury on a person. It can include use of restraints, confinement, and inappropriate use of drugs. The following is considered physical abuse:

- Hitting or striking
- Shoving or pushing
- Shaking
- Burning, mutilation, or maiming
- Throwing objects at the person

- Locking the person in a room

Signs of physical abuse include:

- Fear, paranoia, and/or depression
- Heightened anxiety or discomfort around the suspected abuser
- Unexplained wounds such as bruises, cuts, burns, welts, and scratches
- Unexplained sprains, dislocations, and broken bones
- Rope burns on the wrists, ankles, and around the neck
- Torn clothing and broken glasses, hearing aids, or other damaged or broken devices such as canes or walkers
- Spouse or primary caregiver refuses to allow anyone to see the victim alone
- Unusual covering up with extra clothing such as scarfs, hats, and long-sleeved sweaters

Sexual abuse includes sexual touching or activity without a person's consent. Sexual abuse also includes forcing the person to read or watch pornographic material, to watch live sex acts, or forcing the person to undress in front of others. Signs of sexual abuse include:

- Venereal disease or genital infections
- Unusual vaginal or anal bleeding
- Bloody underclothing
- Bruising around the genitals and breasts

1.3 Neglect and abandonment

Neglect and abandonment is the most common form of elder abuse. A person who is neglectful may refuse to provide the basics such as health care, food and water, clothing, shelter, and other basic necessities. This type of abuse can be intentional or unintentional. In the case of unintentional abuse, the caregiver or spouse may be in denial that the person needs a certain level of care. Neglect is the failure or refusal to provide caregiving obligations.

Signs of neglect:

- Malnutrition, dehydration, and unexplained weight loss
- Untreated bedsores or other medical conditions

- Unsanitary living conditions (e.g., filthy bedding and clothing)

- Desertion of the person in a public place or left home alone locked in a room

- Unsafe living conditions (e.g., no power, heat, or running water, fire hazards, hoarding environment)

- Lack of help in regards to personal hygiene such as he or she is not cleaned after a meal or the person is not bathed regularly

- Refusal to take the person to medical appointments or if an emergency occurs, refusing to take the person to the hospital

- Not giving the person the proper medication or dosage

- Not providing assistance with basic necessities

1.4 Financial abuse

Financial abuse is any unauthorized use of a person's funds, property, and identity theft. It also may include manipulation or exploitation of the elderly person's money and assets. Dishonest use of someone else's money or property or failing to provide for the elderly person with his or her money is considered financial abuse.

Always remember that the elderly person's money and assets are his or hers *not* yours or anyone else's. This person worked hard throughout his or her life and may have saved a significant amount of money to help care for him or her during his or her senior years.

Chapter 6 goes into more detail about strangers who are trying to con or defraud an elderly person. This section describes financial abuse by spouses, friends, family, and hired caregivers.

Financial abuse includes:

- Using the elderly person's personal checks, bank accounts, and credit cards for personal use by someone else

- Stolen cash, personal items, household goods, and income checks

- Forgery

- Identity theft

- Forcing the person to sign over property, vehicles, or other assets

- Misusing a Power of Attorney (or similar document)

- Making the person update his or her will or sign legal documents

Signs of financial abuse:

- Unexplained changes to banking habits and unauthorized ATM withdrawals

- Updates to the person's will, which mainly benefits the suspected financial abuser

- Reduction in cash flow or missing income checks

- Transfer of assets without the involvement of the elderly person

- Signatures on checks and legal documents that do not match the elderly person's signature

- New credit cards arriving in the mail

2. Report Elder Abuse

You must report elder abuse to the authorities and remove the person from the abusive situation. However, it is complicated and there isn't always a quick resolution. You also have to consider the mental stability of the person you are removing from the abusive situation.

You should contact social services, your parent's doctor, the police, and anyone else that can help remove your parent from the abusive situation.

Every state in the US does have toll-free hotlines that deal with elder abuse. The National Council on Child Abuse & Family Violence includes a list of elder abuse hotlines at www.nccafv.org/state_elder_abuse_hotlines.htm#al.

In Canada, you can find some of the provincial and territory contact numbers at this link: www.seniors.alberta.ca/services_resources/elder-abuse/Fact7_WEAAD_E.pdf. You can also contact CARP, a group that is dedicated to advocating for seniors: www.carp.ca.

3. Spousal Abuse

Spousal abuse towards a person with Alzheimer's is a very real topic that is not discussed enough — if it is discussed at all. Everyone who deals with Alzheimer's is willing to discuss caretaker's abusing people with AD or children abusing their parents due to caretaker burnout, but when it comes to the topic of a spouse belittling or physically hurting a person with AD, the information falls into a gray zone.

I found it very frustrating researching this chapter because no one was willing to give me an "expert" opinion to put on record or any definitive advice. I was told over and over again that every situation is different.

While I do agree that every situation is different, the bottom line is there are spouses who verbally, mentally, and/or physically abuse and just because a person with AD has cognitive impairments, it doesn't mean the situation should be tip-toed around or avoided all together.

Because spousal abuse is considered "domestic" it is often an area where no one wants to get involved. It can become more complicated in blended families because children can be accused by a stepparent that they are interfering because they have "never liked" the stepparent and the children are therefore taking advantage of the mentally incompetent parent.

Unfortunately when there is abuse, especially with people suffering from AD, there is a level of codependency between the abused and the abuser. This becomes a bigger problem when it is between an abused AD person and their significant other. The abused person may believe they are being taken care of financially when in reality they may be taken advantage of. It may be hard to separate the abused person from the abuser because of the AD person's fragile state of mind and this codependency aspect. The person may not understand he or she is being abused and therefore he or she may fight you when you try to remove him or her from the situation. If this is your situation, you may need to contact a counselor, psychiatrist, family therapist, or doctor to help you. You may also need to involve the police.

If the person is married to the abuser, divorce may no longer be an option because the person with AD may have already been declared mentally incompetent and therefore, unable to legally sign divorce papers. A guardian or representative may find it hard to file a divorce action because divorce matters are considered too personal to file actions on behalf of people who are mentally incompetent. If your parent is married to an abuser and you are trying to remove him or her from the situation, you should contact an attorney who specializes in Elder Law.

Unfortunately, in many jurisdictions mentally incompetent people are unable to commence a divorce action. In the South Carolina case of Murray v. Murray, 310 S.C. 335, 426 S.E.2d 781 (1993) a son was the guardian of his father and the father's wife was requesting one-third of the husband's property and $400 per month in support. The son filed a divorce action and won, but then it was overturned "because there was no specific legislation authorizing the filing of a divorce action by an incompetent person, and a divorce matter is too personal, a divorce action cannot be maintained unless the plaintiff is capable of exercising reasonable judgment as to his personal decisions, is able to understand the nature of the action, and is able to express unequivocally a desire to dissolve the marriage."[1] The divorce action was denied.

1 Mentally Incompetent Spouses as Parties to Divorce Actions, National Legal Research Group, Inc.

There have been some cases where the AD person was granted a divorce that was petitioned for with the help of a guardian, but they were not easily won battles. The cases went through dismissals, retrials, granting of divorces, overturned decisions, and then granting divorces again. Depending on the jurisdiction where you file an action, it may be easier to gain a legal separation as opposed to a divorce. Again, contact an attorney who specializes in Elder Law.

4. A Personal Story of Emotional Abuse and Neglect

A few years ago, I got a call from someone in California telling me that my aunt and uncle, who lived in Bakersfield, were being abused by their caretaker. By the time I was able to travel to California, it was too late. Everything, including my aunt and uncle's home, personal items, and even their clothes were either sold or discarded. In the end, they were literally left with only the clothes on their bodies.

My aunt and uncle both survived the ordeal, but they had been drugged and physically mistreated to the point where they had to be placed in long-term care homes. It was a heartbreaking situation that caused long-term mental trauma for both my aunt and uncle.

It also caused long-term financial problems because the abuser had opened and maxed out credit cards and got loans in my aunt's name. To this day, my aunt still receives calls from collection agencies.

I can't emphasize enough that if you feel your loved one is being taken advantage of, investigate the situation right away. From the time I got the call to the moment I arrived in California, not even two months had passed. In that time, the abuser got wind of me investigating the situation. The con artist moved quickly to sell my aunt and uncle's home, their personal possessions and then she disappeared. The police were never able to find the person who ruined my aunt and uncle's lives.

The following is another story based on true events; however, names and details have been altered to protect the parties involved.

Mary, who was diagnosed with Alzheimer's, was not married to her boyfriend of 20 years. She was living in a situation of mental and verbal abuse as well as neglect. The boyfriend, John, didn't seem to realize he was an abuser; he came from a big family who yelled and intimidated to get their way. However, it didn't excuse his behavior or the fact it was detrimental to Mary's already fragile state of mind. Mary explained to her children that yelling was the worst thing for her because it made her agitated and stressed, which led her to be more forgetful which caused her boyfriend to yell more thinking she couldn't hear him.

John liked to be in control. He became embarrassed to take Mary out in public and he insisted she stay home and "safe." She was no longer "allowed" to go out and see friends or neighbors, which produced an environment of isolation. A person with AD needs social engagement for many reasons such as to feel purpose and mental stimulation. It has been well documented that social engagement is good for a person with AD while social isolation can make the situation worse, often progressing the disease more rapidly.

Mary's children ran into the socio-cultural norm that emotional abuse by a significant other (i.e., spouse or common-law partner) is a sensitive topic that should be dealt with internally by the family; in other words, it was a private matter. They talked to medical professionals but no one would give them specific advice about what to do to remove their mother from the situation. The children were told over and over, "it's difficult when it comes to family" or "it's hard to say what the right answer is because every situation is different."

Mary became sick with pneumonia and was too sick to inform her children. One of the children, Jane, came by for an unscheduled visit and discovered her mom could barely walk. Mary was in the middle of trying to do laundry for John. Jane was alarmed at her mom's weak state and immediately bundled Mary into some warm clothes and drove her to the hospital.

While they were waiting in the emergency room, Mary told Jane that she had asked John to take her to the hospital but he refused because he felt she was only suffering from a mild flu. Any logical person would have known that she wasn't suffering from the flu but a severe sickness that needed to be medically treated immediately. By him refusing to take her to the hospital, he was neglecting her needs.

The next day, Jane made arrangements to move Mary into her home. She had talked to the emergency room doctor and he agreed that she wasn't getting proper care in her current home.

Jane spent the next couple of months with the help of her siblings, nursing her mom back to health. The boyfriend called on occasion to ask how she was doing and when she would be returning to live with him. He never once visited her, and Jane noticed that every conversation revolved around John and how he needed her mother to take care of him.

When Mary was well enough to talk on the phone, she would talk to John when he called. However, Jane noticed that after the phone calls her mom was moody and disoriented. Jane didn't want to invade her privacy by picking up the phone and listening to what John was saying to Mary, but she was able to catch key words from the conversation and discovered John was pressuring her to move back home with him.

Mary was in the mid-stages of Alzheimer's, which meant she could no longer travel on her own without getting lost and confused. John would try to convince her to take the bus or an airplane by herself to go back to him. He made her feel guilty every time he talked to her, which increased Jane's worries that Mary would wander.

Finally, one day Mary opened up to Jane and told her about one disturbing conversation in which John said, "I'm calling your old friends to see if any want to come and live with me. I might as well get a new girlfriend since you are not coming back." He also added that he called a few of his former girlfriends to see if they were interested in getting back together. Emotionally he was hurting her by using guilt and threats to bully her to return to his home.

John and Mary had a dog that Mary loved very much. One day John called to say he was going to put down her dog since she wasn't there to care for it. Again, he was making her feel guilty for not being there. His cruelty towards Mary seemed to have no end.

When Mary had fully recovered from the illness, Jane took her back to John's for a final "closure" visit and also to pack up the rest of Mary's things. When John opened the door to her, he turned around and walked up the stairs away from her with no greeting or hug or any sign of affection. Mary was hurt as she asked, "What? No hug?"

Mary realized staying with Jane was a safe and better environment for her. However, she wanted Jane talk to John and to explain to him about Alzheimer's and that she would never get better. Jane brought pamphlets she had gathered from her local Alzheimer Society and for an hour she tried to explain the disease to him but he continued to change the subject to him and his sore ankle or his loneliness or his "this or that." Jane would let him speak briefly and then she would politely change the subject back to the topic of Alzheimer's. Mary gave personal examples to coincide with the literature Jane was reading to him. At the end, all he said was, "Are you done?" After he left the room Mary said, "I'm not sure how much of that got through to him." As Jane was to discover later when she left them alone, none of it had sunk in.

Against Jane's better judgment, she gave her mom and John some alone time but she always stayed within hearing distance. Every time she left them alone he would begin his propaganda of how she should be there for him and that Jane was turning Mary against him. To be clear, Jane never once told Mary she couldn't talk to John or visit him, and she was very careful to not say anything bad about him to her mother.

After the third "alone" conversation, Jane had had enough and she interrupted the conversation. John began yelling at Jane and instead of yelling back, she said calmly, "You do not yell at me, especially in front of my mother, and you will never raise your voice to my mother again." If he had listened to what she had read to him from the Alzheimer's literature earlier, one of the topics was not yelling at or in front of someone who has AD because it has such a negative effect on the person.

After the trip, Mary was in a rotten mood for two weeks. Jane kept careful track of Mary's mood swings and triggers. As soon as Mary snapped out of the bad mood, John called and then Jane had another three days of misery.

Jane contacted people in her medical support network and her question was, "Would it be more detrimental to Mary to end the phone calls from John or would it be better to let him keep calling and emotionally abusing her?" Mary had been with John for 20 years and Jane and her siblings didn't know how much control he had over her until she was living with Jane. Mary's mood swings were negatively affecting Jane and her family as well as her mom's well-being.

Mary's anxiety levels increased every time she had to talk to John. She would rarely call him, but Jane figured that was because she never liked using the phone even before she had AD. But looking back, Jane wondered if it was because Mary just didn't want to talk to John anymore but she didn't know how to stop his calls without hurting his feelings. Mary was once a strong and independent woman that wouldn't have taken this abuse.

Jane explained again to Mary's doctor that the anxiety Mary suffers is triggered by John's calls. The doctor finally said he wasn't opposed to Jane blocking John's number so he could no longer call her. She also consulted a psychiatrist and he agreed "off the record" that stopping the calls was probably for the best in her situation.

The result? Mary's mood swings decreased and she no longer thought about John because he was no longer calling to remind her of how guilty she felt for having to leave him because of her disease. However, she still talked about her dog, so Jane would pull out the photo albums, minus pictures of John and go through the dog pictures, reminiscing about the good times Mary remembered with her favorite dog.

CHAPTER 10
Self-Care for the Caregiver

"Forty percent to seventy percent of family caregivers have clinically significant symptoms of depression with about a quarter to half of these caregivers meeting the diagnostic criteria for major depression."[1]

ZARIT, S. (2006)

No matter who you are, you are not a superhero! You will become burned out even just from hanging out with your parent for many days in a row. It can be taxing on the body and mind always worrying about the care of someone you love. It's important to take time for yourself away from everyone. It is said that caregivers are the secondary victims of Alzheimer's disease.

According to a 2003 National Alliance for Caregiving/AARP survey "nearly one in four of the caregivers of people with Alzheimer's disease and other dementias provide 40 hours a week or more of care. Seventy-one percent sustain this commitment for more than a year, and 32 percent do so for five years or more."

Christine Ratkai has worked in child and youth care for 14 years. She said that when she was in college, the professors "stressed the importance of self-care when working with high risk, highly dependent persons." Ratkai added, "At the time I was young and did not quite see the

---

1 Zarit, S. (2006). Assessment of Family Caregivers: A Research Perspective. In Family Caregiver Alliance (Eds.), Caregiver Assessment: Voices and Views from the Field. Report from a National Consensus Development Conference (Vol. II) (pp. 12-37). San Francisco: Family Caregiver Alliance.

importance of true self-care. I was wrong and I have learned the valuable lesson of how truly important self-care really is.

"When working with people, be it ill, highly dependent, or behavioral, it is very important for the caregiver to look after one self. My thought at the time was that I do give myself self-care. I go out with friends, read, take hot baths, and generally I practice some form of self-care. We all do things that we enjoy. But what I was missing was how truly important it was to look after my personal self-care.

"When working, everything becomes about the person you are looking after, all his or her care, food, appointments, chores, discipline, entertainment, all aspects of that person's life is your responsibility. Not to mention your own personal expectations from your family at home.

"In my own personal experience, good self-care took some time to actually grasp. Self-care is more about taking actual time for you, being honest with yourself when you are tired and can't take much more. Self-care needs to be done before you get sick. (Often this requires one to look after one self and too late in the game.) Self-care can be done daily, or it can be taking an entire day to yourself. Self-care is about a person being selfish to degree, which is very difficult for caregivers to do.

"The goal to good self-care, is a daily check-in with yourself to see where you're at. A ten-minute walk will help you rejuvenate, a yoga class, a run, an hour of TV, cuddles with your pet, crafting, or maybe you need a weekend away. You need to be the one in charge of yourself and not to expect others to notice when it seems you have had enough and need the break. Don't be afraid to ask for help and to let people know that you need a break. In the end there is only one of you, and you need to look after that person, which is *you*."

Caregiving can be a full-time job so if you already have a paid job, you may need to talk to your manager and ask if you can take some time off or have more flexibility with your schedule. In the US, there is a federal law that allows employees up to 12 weeks of unpaid time off to care for a close family member. This law is under the *Family and Medical Leave Act*.

If you are part of the "sandwich generation" like Sheila is, you will need to balance taking care of small children and/or teenagers and your parent as well as holding down a full-time job, attending your children's sports and recreational activities, and trying to keep up with your own life.

1. Signs of Caregiver Burnout

As a caregiver, you may feel overwhelmed at times; however, if you are constantly feeling overwhelmed, it is time to ask for help. You need to eat well, exercise regularly, and get enough rest in order to be a good caregiver.

If you need a break, don't be afraid to admit it. Caregiving is hard work so having a day off can go a long way to keeping you healthy. Caregivers who get help are less likely to burnout, and they are better at providing long-term care for their loved one.

Warning signs that you are burning out:

- Emotional lows and highs
- Feeling isolated
- Short temper
- Low energy
- Feeling tired all the time
- Insomnia

2. Take Care of Yourself

You need to take time for yourself away from caregiving duties. Yoga and meditation are good activities to quiet your mind from stress and concentrate on your inner self. Here are some ways to help care for yourself:

- You must take care of yourself. It's not selfish. If you are healthy, you can take better care of your loved one.
- Ask for help from others.
- Keep some of your independence and do activities that don't involve your loved one.
- Express yourself and the emotions you are going through to a close friend, family member, or therapist.
- Do not let others manipulate you through guilt.
- Forgive yourself for your shortcomings and remind yourself that you are doing the best you can for yourself and for your loved one.
- Compliment yourself on doing a good job.
- Find resources in your area to help you take some of the pressure off yourself.
- Humor can help you get through some of the worst times.

Caregiving can be rewarding so consider the positives of being a caregiver:

- A chance to develop a strong relationship with your parent.

- Gives you an opportunity to give back to the parent who raised you.

- Gain new friendships through caregiver support networks.

- Enjoy living in the moment and sharing those good times with your loved one.

- Build memories to cherish after your loved one is gone.

Most people feel they don't have time to exercise but even a walk or run will help you gain more energy and feel better about yourself. Doing a solo physical activity may be just what you need to reduce caregiver stress.

One of the activities I feel is most helpful for me is getting together once a month with my good friends Jocelyn, Janet, and Trudy. Those three ladies give me hours of laughter, which is something I need when I'm feeling overwhelmed. We never discuss anything too serious, instead we enjoy some wine, laughing, and telling funny stories.

3. Get Help

You can find help from community organizations, religious groups, family, friends, or even neighbors. You can contact a local Community Care Access Center, Home Care, or Veterans' Affairs for information on activities your parent can attend without you.

When others offer to help you, say yes because if others are noticing you need help, you are getting close to reaching the burning out stage. Deciding what you need help with may be hard because you may be so overwhelmed you don't know where to begin. Make a list and add to it whenever you think of something. If someone offers help, show him or her the list and let the person pick an item or two that he or she feels comfortable doing for you. For example, taking your parent to an appointment or picking up some items at the store.

Look into placing your parent in an adult day program or respite care. Respite care provides short-term, temporary relief for caregivers, with the parent staying in a facility for a few days while the caregivers take time for themselves to rest and relax. There are many wonderful programs that you can use to help give yourself some alone time.

You may need to hire a caregiver to come into your home a few times a week so you can get important errands done or go to appointments without your parent.

3.1 Join a support group

A support group for AD caregivers can help you feel less isolated. By sharing your problems with others in a similar situation you will find that releasing this information in a supportive atmosphere can help you feel lighter and better about what is going on in your life. Venting your emotions in this supportive atmosphere can also give you stress relief. Sometimes the best resources are other people who are going through a similar situation to your own.

Joining a caregiver group or AD support group can give you new ideas and provide you with effective ways to cope with your parent's disease. You will also find current information about community resources for your parent as well as information about respite care.

A good support group can be a safe environment with like-minded individuals. You can feel comfortable laughing at the absurdities of life without being judged. You can cry or complain knowing that there are others in the room who are going through a similar situation. Sometimes those who don't understand Alzheimer's may judge you on how you take care of your parent; being in a support group means you won't be judged but instead encouraged to stay strong.

If there is a problem that you can't figure out when it comes to caring for your parent, a support group can give you suggestions or examples of what others have done to deal with certain situations.

Resources

Alzheimer's Disease

Alzheimer Society (Canada)

The Alzheimer Society has many informative brochures, booklets, and videos.

www.alzheimer.ca

Alzheimer's Association (USA)

www.alz.org

Alzheimer's Foundation of America

www.alzfdn.org

US Department of Health and Human Services

www.alzheimers.gov

Legal and Advocacy

AARP (American Association of Retired Persons)

www.aarp.org

Canadian Anti-Fraud Centre

www.phonebusters.com/english/reportit_howtoreportfraud.html

CARP (Canadian Association of Retired Persons)

www.carp.ca

Elder Law Answers

This website has a search feature that will help you find an Elder Law Attorney in the United States.

www.elderlawanswers.com/elder-law-attorneys

National Academy of Elder Law Attorneys, Inc. (NAELA)

NAELA is a professional association of attorneys who are dedicated to improving the quality of legal services provided to seniors.

www.naela.org

Caregiver Information and Support

BrightFocus Foundation

www.brightfocus.org

Canadian Caregiver Coalition

www.ccc-ccan.ca

Eldercare Locator

www.eldercare.gov

Family Caregiver Alliance (FCA)

US National Center on Caregiving

www.caregiver.org

Victorian Order of Nurses (VON)

VON put together the following website to help people find advice and resources for caregivers.

caregiver-connect.ca

We Care

Home Health Services

www.wecare.ca

Senior Health

The Alzheimer's Store
This online store sells many wonderful Alzheimer related items.
www.alzstore.com

Johns Hopkins Health Alerts
www.johnshopkinshealthalerts.com/reports/prescriptiondrugs/3363-1.html

Medicare
www.medicare.gov

NIH Senior Health
www.nihseniorhealth.gov

US Administration on Aging (AoA)
www.aoa.gov

Miscellaneous

Emergency Medical Services (EMS) Foundation
For more information about the Capsule of Life® program.
www.emsfoundation.ca

Kids Health
This link provides you with information on how to explain Alzheimer's disease to children.
kidshealth.org/kid/grownup/conditions/alzheimers.html

National Association of Senior Move Managers (NASMM)
nasmm.com

Books

Caregiver's Guide for Canadians, by Rick Lauber

Protect Your Elderly Parents, by Lynn Butler

Still Alice, by Lisa Genova

Alzheimer's Planner for Caregivers

If you would like to build your own *Alzheimer's Planner for Caregivers*, go to www.self-counsel.com/updates/alz/check13.html to download the online kit. It includes forms similar to those described in Chapter 3 as well as bonus forms. Get organized and stay organized!

- Birthdays and Anniversaries
- Caregiver Stress Test
- Debt Tracker
- Doctor's Appointment Notes
- Family Medical History
- Financial Abuse Checklist
- Financial Updates
- Finding an Elder Law Attorney
- Home Safety Checklist
- Important Information
- Income Information

- Medical Contacts
- Medical Devices and Special Needs
- Medicine and Allergy Information
- Monthly Expenses
- Personal Contacts
- Record of Surgeries and Hospital Stays
- Researching Adult Day Programs
- Researching Long-Term Care Homes
- Resources
- Special Events